RESTLESS LEGS SYNDROME

Relief and Hope for Sleepless Victims
of a Hidden Epidemic

ROBERT H. YOAKUM

A Fireside Book
Published by Simon & Schuster
New York   London   Toronto   Sydney

FIRESIDE
Rockefeller Center
1230 Avenue of the Americas
New York, NY 10020

Copyright © 2006 by Robert H. Yoakum
All rights reserved,
including the right of reproduction
in whole or in part in any form.

FIRESIDE and colophon are registered trademarks
of Simon & Schuster, Inc.

For information regarding special discounts for bulk purchases,
please contact Simon & Schuster Special Sales at
1-800-456-6798 or business@simonandschuster.com.

Designed by William Ruoto

Manufactured in the United States of America

10   9   8   7   6   5   4   3   2   1

Library of Congress Cataloging-in-Publication Data is available.

ISBN-13: 978-0-7432-8068-6
ISBN-10:   0-7432-8068-7

To my mother, Eunice A. Yoakum, who died at 101 in 1998, and who suffered from restless legs syndrome for as long as she could remember.

Also, to Pickett Guthrie and Virginia Wilson. For several years these two women devoted most of their waking hours to increasing the awareness and improving the treatment of RLS.

Finally, to the many other volunteers, especially hardworking doctors on the Medical Advisory Board and Scientific Advisory Board of the Restless Legs Syndrome Foundation. Of the devoted volunteers, no one has done more than Robert Waterman, architect of much that has been accomplished. I wish I had the space to praise adequately all the medical pioneers whose research, much of it financially unrewarding, saved nightwalkers untold hours of agony. In some cases they saved lives.

A NOTE TO READERS

CONTENTS

RESTLESS
LEGS
SYNDROME

INTRODUCTION

And miles to go before I sleep,
And miles to go before I sleep.

—ROBERT FROST

"Night Walkers" was the headline I used back in 1994 for an article about restless legs syndrome (RLS) in *Modern Maturity* magazine (since renamed *AARP The Magazine*). The editor's subhead was "Do your legs seem to have a life of their own? Your torment has a name."[1] As an RLS sufferer, I was well suited to write about this odd-sounding illness that is characterized by an urge to move the legs, particularly when at rest. To the editors' astonishment, and mine, more than 40,000 readers wrote to the RLS Foundation. Nearly all expressed relief at discovering that their affliction was real and that they were not alone. Many recounted tales of heartache, triumph, and occasionally, tragedy. They described having to endure sometimes intense creepy-crawly feelings in their legs. They wrote about coping with the profound sleep deprivation that accompanies severe RLS. Some were unable to travel, go to the movies, or even sit still long enough to have dinner with their family. Others lost jobs, were ridiculed or even abandoned by their families. Still others considered self-mutilation and suicide. Readers felt that seeing their experience in print legitimized years of suffering, and their gratitude was affecting. "I cried as I read it." "Thank God I'm not crazy!" "Now I know I'm not the only one." "Finally someone will believe me." "I never knew it had a name." "People just don't understand." "I've been to doctors everywhere for this condition." "I've suffered for years." "Nights are hell." And, from Shirley Pourciau of Jarreau, Louisiana, "Even a year later I thank God for the article."

It is rare for writers to obtain evidence that their words have actually helped. Thousands of letters were generated by the fact that no one—not even the few neurologists who had studied RLS—had realized there were so many nightwalkers. At the time, we had not yet learned that *at least* 12 million Americans—about the same number who have diabetes and five times the number who have Parkinson's disease—suffer from it. And the number may be as high as 40 million.

On *Modern Maturity*'s index page we used a line that has since been quoted in other articles about RLS: "The most common disease you've never heard of." Indeed, most physicians had little or no familiarity with restless legs syndrome. How could such a common disorder be so unknown? One reason is the grossly inadequate amount of time given to the study of sleep in general in medical schools. (RLS, although not solely a sleep disorder but rather a neurologic movement disorder, generally disrupts sleep.) Also, it is an unfortunate fact that doctors rarely ask patients about sleep, and self-conscious patients rarely bring up the subject. Further, when patients do describe the weird sensations that can keep them awake at night, their doctors often wrongly attribute the symptoms to insomnia, stress, depression, muscle cramps, nervous or psychiatric conditions, or aging. Only now are medical professionals beginning to recognize restless legs syndrome for what it is—a sensori-motor disease from which, at least for now, relief can be obtained only through movement or medication.

Although the epidemic of restless legs was obscure back in 1994, in the new millennium the disease has become increasingly better known. Indeed, the last decade has seen an explosion of interest in and information about RLS. Hundreds of scientific articles have appeared in medical journals such as *Sleep, Neurology, Sleep Medicine, Movement Disorders,* and, in the May 2003 issue, a major review in the *New England Journal of Medicine.*[2] Mainstream media have carried many stories on RLS, including news segments on ABC and NBC. Articles about RLS have appeared in major newspapers, including the *New York Times,* the *Boston Globe,* and the *Washington Post.* Jane Brody of the *New York Times* has written two columns on the subject, as has the nationally syndicated medical writer Dr. Peter Gott.

Centuries passed with no increase in either understanding or treatment of RLS, but recently the pace of technological advances in RLS research has been swift. None of the earlier researchers would have predicted that in the year 2005 greatly improved medications would be available. For example, in that year, the Food and Drug Administration approved the GlaxoSmithKlein drug ropinirole (Requip), as appropriate for RLS. The marketing of Requip, which is sure to be followed by FDA approval of other medications for the treatment of RLS, marks a huge advance in research. Only a short time ago—within the last half century—RLS and periodic limb movements (PLM) medications moved from being unknown even in neurological laboratories, to the front pages of medical journals and prominent slots in national and international conferences.

That many RLS victims can now sleep better, even if not well, is thanks in part to devoted researchers, mostly academic, who worked into the nights.

While awareness has improved, millions continue to suffer from RLS. Cases range from mild (people shift uncomfortably while sitting in a theater or airplane) to severe (people are forced to get out of bed and walk, sometimes until dawn, by an intolerable sensation in the legs). Even today many people with RLS have yet to identity their affliction.

I'd had restless legs for many years but, not suspecting that it was an identifiable disease, complained only to my mystified wife. However, the symptoms got much worse in February of 1991 after I underwent an operation at Johns Hopkins University Hospital to remove a cancerous prostate.

The operation was a success, but while still in the hospital I was plagued as never before by both restless legs and another condition known as PLM. Unknown to me, progress on both disorders was being made by neurologists in that very same hospital. Not long after the operation I received a copy of the *Hopkins Medical News* and was riveted by an excellent description of my tortures in an article entitled "Rest for the Weary." I recognized my enemies immediately. They were called RLS and PLM. The article cited Dr. David Buchholz, associate professor of neurology at Johns Hopkins:

People with restless legs syndrome get what Buchholz calls "creepy-crawly" sensations in their legs when they lie in bed and try to fall asleep. The feeling, centered mostly in the calf muscles, is "very distressing, and it drives people crazy to try to lie still." Moving—pacing, massaging or stretching the muscles, or bicycling the legs in bed—provides temporary relief. But then it comes right back as they try to lie still again. It's a plague for the people who have it.[3]

I read on with increasing excitement. Was relief at hand? Thank God, this affliction has a name and I'm not alone! "The disorder is not rare," Buchholz is quoted as saying. "And it may run in families."

I then experienced epiphany number two: so this is what tortured my mother at night? When I questioned her, I learned that both my parents suffered from RLS. The odds were high that I would inherit the disease.

I immediately shared what I learned with my doctors, Richard Collins, the superb diagnostician who discovered my prostate cancer, and Britain Nicholson, chief medical officer of Massachusetts General Hospital in Boston, neither of whom had heard of RLS. Both enlisted in my search for more information.

It's almost certain that I had PLM twitches before the radical prostatectomy, according to my medical advisers, but I hadn't been aware of them. It's possible that the operation triggered PLM but more likely that previously mild symptoms became more severe.

When the surgical residents arrived at 6:30 a.m., I complained that restless, twitching legs had kept me awake. They nodded sympathetically but did nothing. After my third protest, they prescribed a benzodiazepine, Ativan, designed to slow down the central nervous system ("for spasms," it said on the bottle), and Tylox (oxycodone and acetaminophen), which is given for postoperative pain and sometimes prescribed for RLS. The Tylox should have helped, but I later learned that tricyclic antidepressants, one of which, Elavil, I was taking for postoperative depression, can not only exacerbate RLS but actually cause it. Ironically, it may be that the depression for which I was taking Elavil came not only from the operation but also from sleep deprivation caused by RLS—which was being exacerbated by the antidepressant.[4]

This book is for all my fellow sufferers and those who care for them.

Every reader is likely to know a nightwalker. Some victims have had RLS since infancy. Others have developed it much later in life, first noticing symptoms when they have been sitting still for a long time, or when, after lying down to sleep, they find themselves impelled to move their legs. We may not even know that someone in our life has RLS, for though it's both ancient and common, the disease has long been overlooked, and its victims have often been isolated, neglected, and misunderstood. I hope to show people with RLS that they are not alone, not insane, and not beyond help. Correctly identifying the problem is an enormous first step toward getting relief. Most of the writers who responded to my "Night Walkers" article, never having seen their disease described before, were ecstatic, some crediting the article with saving their lives. One such thankful person was Nancy Lee Hixson, who had suffered from RLS all her life, but only learned there was a name for her problem when she stumbled on my magazine article about it at age fifty.

Scores of doctors, from here and abroad, helped me write this book. Aid came from researchers and clinicians, especially neurologists, who are in the vanguard of the fight to understand and treat RLS. Still, many health care workers are unaware of RLS. We need a strong effort to educate the medical community as well as the general public. Spearheading this movement is the RLS Foundation, which has as its objectives increasing awareness of the disease, developing treatments, and, through research, finding a cure.

This book emerged from the anguish and self-pity I felt on hundreds of nights, and also from empathy with all those who have suffered even more than I. It is my humble hope that this book will shed considerable light on a disease that has often involved much darkness.

CHAPTER 1

Yes, It Is a Real Disease

The miserable have no other medicine, but only hope.

—WILLIAM SHAKESPEARE, *MEASURE FOR MEASURE*

The word *nightwalkers* describes people (like me) who are forced to endure profoundly disagreeable creepy-crawly symptoms in their legs that can be relieved only by movement or medication. Walking is the method most commonly used, and since the restless limbs suffer more at night, the severely afflicted may have to walk all night long. Hence *nightwalkers*.

The severity of symptoms ranges from mild (uncomfortable and intermittent), to moderate, to severe (distressing and daily). Those with the severe form—who have the agony of serious sleep deprivation as well as the discomfort of RLS—have in some cases been driven to suicide.

My RLS eventually became severe: sleep was impossible until daybreak. I spent many dark hours walking. I can testify from experience that the name *restless legs syndrome,* though sounding trivial, does accurately describe the nature of the affliction. Legs, and sometimes arms, demand to be moved.

People with RLS have employed many words in their attempts

to relay their unusual discomfort: "prickly," "jittery," "pulling," "an electrical feeling," "pressure building up," "fidgety," "like thousands of ants crawling inside," "heebie-jeebies," "a deep ache in the bones," "as though a very large spring was coiled inside my legs," "like a cramp that does not fully develop." The character Kramer on the TV sitcom *Seinfeld* said his girlfriend had "jimmy legs," which is probably another way of describing RLS. A psychiatrist with RLS described the sensation as "ineffable," adding, "It's like an itch that you can't scratch," which gives added force to the aphorism that "the severity of an itch is inversely proportional to the ability to reach it."

Since RLS is treatable, though not yet curable, the only way for Kramer's girlfriend to obtain relief is through medication or movement. If she is like most RLS sufferers, her symptoms fluctuate, and she seeks comfort by walking, stretching, rocking, or riding an exercise bicycle.

EARLY WRITING ABOUT RLS

Restless legs syndrome has been around for a long time. An early account of RLS appears in the essay "Of Experience" by French author Michel de Montaigne (1533–92):

That preacher is very much my friend who can oblige my attention a whole sermon through; in places of ceremony, where everyone's countenance is so starched, where I have seen the ladies keep even their eyes so fixed, I could never order it so, that some part or other of me did not lash out; so that though I was seated, I was never settled. As the philosopher Chrysippus' maid said of her master, that he was only drunk in his legs, for it was his custom to be always kicking them about in what place soever he sat; and she said it, when the wine having made all his companions drunk, he found no alteration in himself at all; it may have been said of me from my infancy that I had either folly or quicksilver in my feet, so much stirring and unsettledness there is in them, wherever they are placed.[1]

A British physician, Sir Thomas Willis, was the first medical observer to describe what appears to have been both RLS and PLM:

Wherefore to some, when being a-Bed they betake themselves to sleep, presently in the Arms and Legs, Leapings and Contractions of the Tendons, and so great a Restlessness and Tossings of other Members ensue, that the diseased are no more able to sleep, than if they were in a Place of the greatest Torture.[2]

This account was published in *The London Practice of Physick* in 1683. Note that Willis includes arms in his description. For most people, it's legs that cause discomfort, but scientists prefer the word *limb* because arms can also be involved. An unfortunate small minority of victims suffer from full-body akathisia, which is "a condition of motor restlessness in which there is a feeling of muscular quivering, an urge to move about constantly, and an inability to sit still."[3]

The groundbreaking RLS medical study was done by Karl A. Ekbom, a Swedish neurologist, in 1945. In a systematic and comprehensive report, he defined the clinical features of the syndrome, including familial component, epidemiology, and therapy. After his pioneering research, the disease became known in some circles as *Ekbom's syndrome*. While in some countries, such as England, the name is still used, it was the brilliant doctor himself who coined "restless legs syndrome," and that name stuck.[4]

In the nearly three hundred years between the Willis observation and the clinical studies by Ekbom and others, those who wrote about RLS tended to identify it as a "hysterical" condition. Until well into the twentieth century, RLS was labeled *anxietas tibiarum*, or anxious legs. Only more recently have neurologists begun to realize that we are dealing with a disease of the central nervous system, not a neurosis.

WHAT CAUSES RLS?

Research into the causes of RLS is ongoing but so far has not pinpointed the mechanism underlying the disease. In other words, RLS has no identifiable origin, as, for example, influenza does. It may be that RLS is a final common pathway for multiple causes and mechanisms. Or it may be that victims have an underlying vulnerability that develops in the presence of one or more precipitating factors.

The word *cause* is used here in a loose fashion to mean something that appears to cause or trigger the disagreeable symptoms of RLS.

In nearly half of all cases, RLS is familial, but it may be idiopathic (cause unknown) or related to another condition.

PRIMARY RLS

Primary RLS very often includes a positive family history. Between one-third and one-half of RLS cases are transmitted in a pattern consistent with autosomal dominant traits. (Human traits, including an individual's eye color, hair color, or expression of certain diseases, result from the interaction of one gene inherited from the father and one gene from the mother. In autosomal dominant disorders, the presence of a single copy of a mutated gene may result in the disease. In other words, the mutated gene may dominate or "override" the instructions of the normal gene on the other chromosome, potentially leading to disease expression. Individuals with an autosomal dominant disease trait have a 50 percent risk of transmitting the mutated gene to their children.) There is also some evidence of a recessive inheritance,[5] meaning that RLS cases can be transmitted by the less dominant, or recessive, gene. Primary RLS can also reflect a dopaminergic deficiency, which may result from a malfunction in the brain stem.

SECONDARY RLS

Features of secondary RLS are referred to as *risk factors for RLS* or as *comorbid*—coexisting disease states or disorders that occur *in conjunction with* RLS. Examples include periodic limb movements (PLM), end-stage renal disease (ESRD), early-onset Parkinson's disease, venous insufficiency, diabetes, peripheral neuropathy, rheumatoid arthritis, fibromyalgia, lumbar radiculopathy, third-trimester pregnancy, iron-deficiency anemia, uremia, and attention-deficit/hyperactivity disorder (ADHD). There have been some reports of RLS symptoms resulting from deficiencies of vitamin B_{12}, folate, and magnesium.

RLS can be induced by certain drugs, including all drugs that block the dopamine receptor—including neuroleptics, many antiemetic or antinausea drugs, and metoclopramide (Reglan)—as well as tricyclic antidepressants, selective serotonin reuptake inhibitors, and lithium. Alcohol and caffeine use can also trigger restless legs syndrome.

Another trigger appears to be physical trauma. No formal research supports this conclusion, but anecdotal evidence is strong.

For example, my own experience, and that of many other people with RLS, leads me to believe that the disease occasionally follows or is at least exacerbated by operations, accidents, or other sorts of insults to the body and brain. In my case it was a radical prostatectomy. Others have reported that RLS was brought on or worsened by an accident.

So should I blame the onset of my RLS on the trauma of the operation itself? Or should I blame the use of Elavil afterward, since nearly all antidepressants are contraindicated for RLS victims? Or was it the accumulation of metabolites in the legs from venous congestion—a possible trigger of RLS, according to Ekbom? (I was hurled back into bed and given a blood thinner on what was to have been the day of my discharge. Dangerous blood clots were discovered in the deep vein of my right leg.) The RLS might have been worsened by the trauma of the operation or by the damaged veins, iron deficiency from blood loss, or either all, or none, of the above.

Other triggers guilty of worsening preexisting mild RLS include arthritis of the lumbar region, and spinal surgery. The most common link, according to Dr. Mark Buchfuhrer, of the former Gallatin Medical Clinic in Downey, California, "seems to be with lumbar laminectomy surgery (possibly due to the fact that this is one of the most common back surgeries), but even cervical (neck) surgery seems to be a not uncommon trigger of this type of RLS."

"The differential diagnosis of RLS is usually uncomplicated," Dr. John Winkelman, medical director of the Sleep Health Center at Brigham and Women's Hospital in Boston and former member of the RLS Foundation Medical Advisory Board, wrote in a November 1999 article in *Nephrology News & Issues* magazine:

Some forms of peripheral neuropathy are the most difficult disorders to distinguish from RLS, and in fact the two not infrequently coexist. Painful neuropathy is often a "burning" superficial dysesthesia which is usually unaffected by movement, whereas RLS is more often a "crampy" deep-seated feeling which is relieved by movement. Both can worsen in the evening and night.

Patients with both disorders can be taught to distinguish the two types of discomfort, which can be helpful to the treating physician. Other disorders in the differential include pruritus (which can produce abnormal sensations with restlessness and sleep loss), anxiety, and akathisia (inner restlessness caused by dopaminergic blockers or antagonists).[6]

In his search for the cause of his RLS, Leonard J. Uttal, of Blacksburg, Virginia, believes that he "hit the jackpot."

After trying to get other doctors interested in my RLS, I sought a neurologist with geriatric and psychiatric qualifications on the combined advice from the RLS Foundation and AARP. This gentleman of a doctor spent three hours with me, performed neurological tests, and furnished me with reprints from the literature. He is most conversant with peripheral neuropathy, of which I have a "moderately severe" case and which often is associated with RLS symptoms. Also, together we dug out injuries to my legs I suffered over fifty years ago as a possible cause. Also, since I had heart bypass surgery a year and a half ago, an interrupted blood supply can be a cause, as can some medications. He plans to evaluate everything to try to pinpoint why I have RLS and work from there on. He plans to work with my internist who controls my medications to try to get me off as many as possible. For the first time I feel I am on track, in no small measure due to the RLS Foundation and AARP.

A SOLDIER'S TALE

I was an infantry platoon commander in the Marine Corps. I was twenty-three years old, a lieutenant. Often my platoon would come back from patrols exhausted. We hadn't slept for days. The others would fall asleep on the ground, but I'd be there wiggling around with my restless legs forcing me to stay awake. Sometimes I could doze for maybe half an hour. I never got real sleep. I remember ambush situations where we had to lie there and not move. My life, and the lives of the guys with me, depended on it. My legs desperately needed to move but even the slightest motion could betray our position. It was torture.

This Vietnam veteran, Barry Kowalski, had symptoms of RLS as a child, but they were mild and intermittent. Restless legs syndrome typically worsens with age, and this was certainly the case for this soldier. By the time he was in his early twenties, the RLS was appearing almost nightly and he was forced to seek medical help.

Kowalski turned to several doctors, none of whom were very familiar—if at all— with this disease. Together they experimented with various medications, some of which provided temporary relief. Eventually he would develop a tolerance to the medication and need to take an increased dosage.

Unfortunately, Kowalski's difficulty in finding effective treatment was typical, since at this time very few doctors had even heard of RLS. Indeed, twenty years passed before Kowalski learned that his problem was compounded by PLM, a related disease that causes legs to twitch or jerk about every thirty seconds or so.

Lieutenant Kowalski later became lawyer Kowalski and gained national attention as a prosecutor on the Rodney King case, working for the Civil Rights Division of the Justice Department. In the spring of 1992, after the Los Angeles riots, he went to L.A. to prepare the federal trial.

When I went out to Los Angeles, I knew that my disease had a name, but I hadn't found a drug that helped much. I never got enough sleep. I was in agony from being so tired. Because of RLS, I usually wouldn't get to sleep until three in the morning. And I had to get up at six because of the heavy workload. That went on for months.

Then came the trial and another two months of stultifying fatigue. Those were tense times, and I was totally exhausted when the trial was over. It was a year of hell. When I gave the closing argument in the case, I remember thinking very vividly that I had had only four hours of sleep in the past two days.

In a recent interview, more than ten years after the Rodney King trial, Kowalski said that the intervening years had been bad, not only because of RLS and PLM but because he was still "badly hooked on Klonopin." He stayed on a low dose of the drug because "if I cut it out altogether, I got powerful withdrawal symptoms."

As of this writing, Barry Kowalski takes a potion prescribed by a psychiatric pharmacologist who is learning about RLS. "Now I sleep well, but only after a struggle to get to sleep." Although not cured, he is much better off than he was. As word spreads about RLS, and as treatments continue to improve, it is unlikely that future victims will spend so many difficult years struggling for relief from this trivial-sounding yet serious disease.

HOW COMMON IS IT?

How many people have RLS? Medically, RLS is considered a "common" disorder, as well as an epidemic, since it affects 7 to 15 percent of the northern European and U.S. population. Obtaining precise figures is difficult for a variety of reasons, particularly because a lack of research funds makes undertaking a large epidemiologic study impossible. Suffice to say, though, at least 12 million and up to 40 million Americans suffer from RLS—numbers that are far higher than those for widely known diseases such as diabetes and Parkinson's.[7]

Periodic limb movements (PLM) often coexists with RLS but is a separate affliction that involves leg twitches or jerks that occur about every twenty to forty seconds. PLM is used to describe periodic movement of the limbs while awake or sleeping, and usually in conjunction with RLS. This is not to be confused with PLMS, which is repeated stereotypic movements of the limbs (usually the legs) that occur during sleep. Both are independent of PLMD, or periodic limb movement disorder. The diagnosis of PLMD is made by polysomnography with electromyographic (EMG) recordings from the tibialis anterior muscles. The severity of PLMD is determined by the periodic limb movement index (PLMI), which equals the number of periodic limb movements per hour of sleep. Mild PLMD is defined as 5–25 periodic limb movements per hour of sleep; moderate as 25–50 periodic limb movements per hour of sleep; and severe as more than 50 periodic limb movements per hour of sleep or greater than 25 periodic limb movements associated with arousals per hour of sleep.

The limb movements of PLM are easily measured with monitors; RLS, however, cannot be confirmed by laboratory tests, thus adding to the difficulty of establishing a precise prevalence rate. While RLS keeps people from sleeping at all, PLM keeps people from having sound sleep. According to Dr. Daniel Picchietti, medical director of the Carle Clinic in Urbana, Illinois, "It's a double whammy. RLS affects the quantity of sleep while PLM affects the quality of sleep."

Earlier prevalence studies suffered not only from inadequate funding but also from their dependence on patients' subjective answers to questions. Further, the studies often used minimum frequency criteria, which failed to include many mild, intermittent sufferers.

Here is what we know about the numbers when we extrapolate from available statistics: In the United States and Canada (and probably elsewhere, judging from studies in Italy, Germany, and the United Kingdom), at least 3 percent of adults are fatigued *daily* by RLS and PLM and face each night with fear and despair. They must walk into the night, perhaps until daybreak, to rid themselves of intolerable sensations.

Stanford University researchers led by Dr. William C. Dement, former chair of the National Committee on Sleep Disorders and President of the American Sleep Disorders Association, and Dr. Clete Kushida, chair of the Standards of Practice Committee, American Academy of Sleep Medicine, were startled to see the results of a 1997–98 study they conducted in Moscow, Idaho.[8] It showed that 29.3 percent of the population has symptoms similar to RLS. Intrigued, researchers launched a new study where the RLS prevalence was reported at a more reasonable 15.3 percent.[9]

The National Sleep Foundation conducted a poll in 2005.[10] It found that 25 percent of adults experienced "unpleasant feelings in their legs (such as creepy-crawly or tingling sensations) a few nights a month or more, 15 percent a few nights a week or more," and 8 percent reported these symptoms every night or almost every night. Half of those who described symptoms said they couldn't get a good night's sleep. Nearly 25 percent of respondents over the age of sixty-five reported having symptoms of RLS. A mere 3 percent of those with symptoms said their doctor had told them they had RLS.

The previous NSF polls in 1999, 2000, 2001, 2002, and 2003 had reported almost identical findings, with 57 percent of respondents saying that symptoms kept them from sleeping; only 2 percent were told by a physician that they had RLS.[11]

Restless legs syndrome can seriously disturb daily activities. This fact, and the profound underdiagnosis rate, have recently been confirmed by the largest multinational study to date.[12] The REST (RLS, Epidemiology, Symptoms and Treatment) Study in Primary Care showed that more than half of RLS sufferers (estimated to be one in thirty of all patients seen by the primary care doctors) reported a lack of energy, disturbance of daily activities, difficulty sitting or relaxing, and a tendency to feel depressed or down. One-third of the sufferers said RLS symptoms had a high negative impact on their quality of life, while two-thirds said they had some negative impact.

Many beleaguered nightwalkers, compelled to move, are deprived of sleep every night. Absent proper medical care, the severely afflicted are discouraged and always fatigued. They are also lonely. Yet, in the care of an informed doctor, nearly all would experience some relief. This was the case for a retired aircraft machinist who had struggled with RLS—although he didn't know it as that—for more than twenty years.

"I'm at the edge of a cliff," he told Dr. Philip Becker, president of Sleep Medicine Associates of Texas, "and I'm ready to go over." Sometimes he walked twenty hours a day. Because of worsening RLS, he was able to sleep only three or four hours at daybreak. His suffering was greatly increased because of two heart bypass operations and three joint replacements. He was also taking medications for diabetes and high blood pressure. Other ailments included sleep apnea and mild peripheral neuropathy that caused numbness in his feet. Hoping to alleviate the machinist's severe depression, a family doctor had given him an antidepressant, but as is so often the case with these drugs, it made his RLS worse.

Dr. Becker was able to turn this patient's life around. After a year's treatment, the man was on a new drug, off the antidepressant, and sleeping six or seven hours a night. Dr. Becker may well have saved his desperate patient's life.

As yet Dr. Becker's expertise is not shared by all physicians, but awareness of restless legs syndrome is growing. With progress being made in education and research, many more nightwalkers can now hope to find understanding and, at last, relief.

CHAPTER 2

Eighteen Years:
The Misdiagnosis of RLS

Throw physic to the dogs: I'll none of it.

—WILLIAM SHAKESPEARE, MACBETH

Many millions seek relief from RLS, yet it is routinely underdiagnosed and diagnosed late—taking an average of eighteen years. According to neurologist William Ondo, of Baylor College of Medicine, "RLS is probably the single most misdiagnosed disease—period. Not neurologically, just disease—period. I can't imagine anything else that has a correct diagnosis rate of 30 percent, or an eighteen-year latency to a correct diagnosis." Imagine enduring eighteen distressing years from when symptoms first appear to a correct diagnosis. As sleep expert Dr. William Dement says, "Something has to be done about this terrible disorder. Restless legs syndrome has got to be the biggest completely unaddressed health care priority in America."[1] Indeed, because the medical community has not been adequately informed about restless legs syndrome, and rarely asks patients about sleep, finding helpful medical care has proven a major challenge for nightwalkers.

Some have spent decades and thousands of dollars trying to find out what ails them. At least ten thousand of the letters generated by my *Modern Maturity* article dealt with doctors who had been seen—to no avail—by beleaguered readers. RLS is still so little known that four doctors, hearing a patient describe its symptoms, might—like the four blind men describing an elephant by touch—prescribe four different medications. Since doctors erroneously attribute symptoms to insomnia, stress, depression, muscle cramps, nervous or psychiatric conditions, or aging, the medicines they prescribe are often of little consequence to the RLS sufferer. The most common of these, which have little or no effect, are

The following letter, a classic of its kind, was reprinted in *NightWalkers,* the RLS Foundation's newsletter. It is from Nancy Lee Hixson, of Danville, Ohio.

When I look in a mirror, the tired, nervous, sallow, sunken-eyed, slightly frayed reflection always startles me, for I expect to see someone young, tan, lean, fit, alert. I expect to see my fifty summers reflected there, but instead I see only fifty winters. Why so great a dichotomy? Because the mirror accurately reflects what I've tried so hard to hide, the persistent exhaustion, the relentless frustration, of a half century of undiagnosed and untreated RLS.

The gross pain didn't start until I was ten, in the fifth grade, but school report cards of the four preceding years contain notes from teachers that reflect my earlier symptoms. First grade: "She is a happy child but cannot seem to sit still in class." Second grade: "She seems to have a great deal of difficulty staying in her seat." Third grade: "She is bright and cooperative but can't sit still for more than a few minutes." Fourth grade: "Nancy has ants in her pants."

By fifth grade the school nurse said "growing pains," but it was exasperating, embarrassing, to find I simply *couldn't* sit still and had no *believable* excuse for it. I became a nighttime head-rocker, wearing the hair off the back of my head, and a daytime chair-rocker, for there was some great measure of relief in rocking.

I learned to run, climb, leap, bike, ski, skate, and swim to keep my antsy legs moving, for the activity numbed the pain. But nighttimes, when the world of children stopped and quiet stars watched, I was wrapping my tormented legs with hot towels—in a plastic shower curtain to keep the bed dry.

Teenage years were worse as I shied from overnighters and pajama parties, suffered through the interminable inactivity of movies, theater, and church, and endured the unendurable in school classrooms and college lecture halls. Now, though, neurologists were saying "hysteria."

In my twenties, I faced night classes, activism, a career, motherhood, children's piano/dance/banjo/skating lessons, Scouts, Sunday school, sleepless nights, separate beds, divorce, and pain. The psychologist said "dissociative disorder."

In my thirties, I found a new love (who still valiantly hangs on for a rough ride) and a compassionate MD who prescribed small nightly doses of Percocet, coincidentally one of the drugs of choice for RLS, and I was actively seeking answers in alternative medicine, for by then the psychiatrist was mumbling something about "multiple personalities."

In my forties, there were a few alternative palliatives for the pain, so I tried them all: acupuncture, acupressure, aromatherapy, biofeedback, reflexology, self-hypnosis, homeopathy, massage, ointments, vitamins, oils, and herbals. As a naturopathic physician specializing in poisonous and medicinal plants, I long had been searching their repertoire for pain and spasm relievers. Through careful, persistent experimentation I was able to keep my days livable and my nights just bearable.

Finally, at fifty, by the most obscure coincidence, I found myself in an Ohio State University Medical Center hallway idly thumbing through a battered copy of *Modern Maturity* magazine and I stumbled onto an article about RLS. I nearly sank to my knees right there in the hall to thank God, Allah, Brahma, Buddha, Confucius, Mohammed, and every other entity who may have had a hand in my finding that particular article in a magazine I had never read before that day.

I wept . . . I'm free at last, free at last; thank God Almighty, I'm free at last. Yes, I have RLS. I always knew I had it. I just didn't know what to call it or where to go for help. Please, please, emphasize educating members of the medical and teaching professions so others like me won't lie abed in midnight agony with clenched teeth for forty years of hopeless nights.

aspirin, ibuprofen, and other painkillers; sleeping pills; quinine; tranquilizers; and allergy drugs. Also antidepressants, which not only don't relieve symptoms but can trigger or even aggravate them.

Once thought to be a disease of the elderly, RLS can plague people for decades, beginning in childhood. Health workers and others should be alert to the possibility that youngsters, especially those who have trouble sleeping or sitting still in school, may already be RLS victims.

It was decades before a proper diagnosis was made for Thelma Dean Stewart, of Girard, Illinois. She had had RLS since age sixteen. At seventy-one she wrote:

> I could write a book on my trials and tribulations with the outrageous things different doctors have put me through, hoping to hit on something. All I hear from doctors and nurses is they never heard of RLS. When I had surgery in January, my doctor had to look it up in a book. He was very nice and used the epidural for five days so I could lie in bed. That was the best five days I have had since I was a young girl.

Another patient, Marilyn Culican, of Potomac, Maryland, was told that her symptoms were caused by "some chemical imbalance—or caused by MSG or NutraSweet, both of which have been removed from my diet, to no avail."

George L. Youngren, of Lakewood, Colorado, reported, "I have had [RLS] for at least forty to forty-five years. I have been to at least twenty doctors. . . . There were times I could have committed suicide. I found a neurosurgeon who worked with me for forty-five minutes and said I had RLS. He put me on Klonopin and codeine and in three days the pain just about cleared."

As Mrs. Dewey H. Bennett, of Columbia, Missouri, recalled,

"My own experience with this living nightmare began in 1972. . . . After having run the gamut of specialists of all kinds, tests of all kinds, antidepressants of all names, and having spent four nights at the University of Missouri sleep lab, I believe I finally have an ally and some answers concerning this mysterious torment."

Tommie Hance, of Dallas, Texas, consulted "several doctors but none seem to understand. . . . One doctor said I have arthritis and I will just have to learn to live with it." Another diagnosed severe depression and prescribed an antidepressant. "That pill sent me climbing the walls."

A professor in Whittier, California, not only had trouble finding help for RLS but suffered more on the operating table because her RLS made another condition worse:

I have shared my RLS with every doctor I've seen, no matter what my ailment or the doctor's specialty, including a hypnotist, a psychologist, a chiropractor, podiatrist, dentist, dermatologist, neurologist, orthopedic surgeon, etc., etc. Some were very kind and made suggestions (which didn't help, but they *tried*), while others were so condescending, I cried on the way home. One actually ridiculed me for making the whole thing up. *They just didn't understand!*

A few years ago I had knee surgery. Whatever was in that shot to make me relax had an immediate rebound effect. There was no way I could hold my leg still while the doctor was cutting and stitching. He yelled at me: "Hold still! You're kicking me in the face!" I explained that I had restless legs. His reply: "I can tell you have restless legs. *Hold them still!*" Finally his nurse crawled up on the table and threw herself across my legs, lying there until the surgery was over.

Charles W. Skillas, PhD, of Norcross, Georgia, "spent over $100,000 seeking relief. I have been in and out of sleep centers all over the USA without success. The best that medical science has been able to do for me is to drug me into insensibility to get any sleep. This, of course, then gives rise to addiction and withdrawal."

The good news is that patients can find relief even after decades of medical misguidance. The right doctor and correct diagnosis can change a person's life. Jo Snider, of Austin, Texas, lived with RLS symptoms for twenty years. Then she found effective treatment:

> My depression, anxiety, and physical problems disappeared. For the first time in my entire adult life (I'm fifty-one), I know how normal people live. I go to bed at a reasonable hour, wake refreshed, no longer nap, and look five years younger. I am twice as productive, and I cope with the world, if not totally serenely, at least effectively and calmly. My family has been astonished at the change. For myself, I was surprised to dream, something I hadn't done in years.

"My doctor has literally saved my life," wrote Leona Meyer, of Monango, North Dakota. "I started seeing him several years ago and he hadn't heard of RLS at that time. He has learned a lot since then. He took such an interest in this condition, and made me promise that when I feel suicidal, I will call him first. He has become such a treasured friend."

"IT'S ALL IN YOUR HEAD"

Many restless legs victims have been told by their doctors that they needed psychiatric care. How could any doctor, sworn to do no harm, tell patients with a serious sensorimotor disease that their problem is psychological? That the problem is not with their legs but with their heads? The main reason is ignorance. Failing to learn about RLS in medical school, physicians did, however, learn about the ability of the human mind to imagine afflictions. Lacking a better explanation for vague or odd-sounding complaints like "I have to keep moving around every night because it feels like ants are crawling inside my legs," the uninformed doctor may retreat to neurosis as the explanation.

Indeed, the word *nerves* appears frequently in patients' retelling of their encounters with skeptical doctors. One patient in Ohio, describing her long battle with severe RLS, described how "for years the doctors blamed it on 'nerves, depression.' " That same diagnosis was offered from Michigan to the Middle East. Professor Bernard Katz, from Ramat Aviv, Israel, recounted how "I've suffered with the problem [RLS] for almost fifty years, since my early twenties. I don't know how many different diagnoses I've had, especially by neurologists. . . . I recall my first diagnosis by a neurologist who, after examining X-rays of my head and back, told me I was suffering from hysteria and should see a psychiatrist."

In one sense, the problem actually *is* in the head, because the neurotransmitter dopamine is clearly involved. But dopamine insufficiency isn't what the doctors had in mind when one of them treated Jo Snider, of Austin, Texas, for depression. After a year he recommended "a complete psychiatric evaluation" for Ms. Snider, who sensibly reacted, "I was appalled, but also angry enough to seek another medical opinion and treatment."

John Williams, a former RLS Foundation board member, consulted "two GPs, an orthopedist, two chiropractors, an osteopath, two internists, and five neurologists. One doctor told me to go to a psychiatrist, and I went to one who, after a thousand dollars or so, gave me the startling conclusion that I had repressed rage toward my parents because babies kick when they're mad at their parents."

Gilda Scarangello, of Brooklyn, New York, wrote that she and her husband "both just turned sixty-five and have been RLS sufferers. Several times over the years we have asked the doctors what it was and explained how our sleep was disturbed. The answer was always the same. They would look at our legs and say it was our imagination." Even worse is the outright humiliation experienced by people like Louise M. Scherer, of Indianapolis. "I have been embarrassed, belittled, laughed at by some doctors and nurses, and have even been called a hypochondriac because they refuse to believe that there is such a disease."

Suffering the discomfort of limbs that demand movement, as well as the fatigue that accompanies sleep deprivation, and being unable to find relief or even validation of one's suffering can, in fact, make one question one's own sanity. It is a common experience among nightwalkers: "For years I thought I was crazy."

Sally Franklin, of Gering, Nebraska, took a break from late-night walking to write her story:

> I am writing to you at 1:30 a.m. because of my legs. I went to bed about two hours ago and here I am up again. I would say I am one of the more severe cases but I'm sure everyone that has this feels the same. I have been suffering with RLS for many, many years and have gone to many, many doctors . . . but I get the same answer, "We can't find anything" and of course *I go home thinking that it is all in my head,* but the only problem is that my legs are still driving me crazy.

Some of those misdiagnosed with psychological problems are given antidepressants. Others are given antidepressants because they have, indeed, become depressed as a result of sleep deprivation. Even those prescriptions are a mistake, however, because most antidepressants can make RLS worse.

Advancing age can make it even more difficult for people with RLS to find proper treatment. "I can hardly take this RLS any longer," wrote a ninety-year-old widow who lived alone and suffered from severe RLS. Her doctor "mistook RLS for anxiety and depression" and the woman ended up in a psychiatric ward. Such accounts help explain why awareness is the first objective of the RLS Foundation. Awareness leads to research, which leads to treatment, which will eventually lead to a cure.

American doctors are not alone in diagnosing RLS victims as demented or at least hallucinatory. Responding to the *Modern Maturity* article, Dr. Pasquale Montagna, of the University of Bologna, which boasts one of the world's best research centers for RLS and PLM, observed that although his university did pioneering work with PLM in the 1960s (Dr. Elio Lugaresi made the first polygraphic recordings of nocturnal myoclonus in 1966), the "status" of RLS in Italy "has hardly changed since those early times. RLS is almost never recognized by the family doctor, symptoms usually being ascribed to a nervous disposition, to arthritis, or vascular leg problems." Dr. Montagna had been called as a neurologist consultant "to see patients thought to be crazy or demented because they were unable to stay through a dialytic procedure for kidney failure. They just had severe RLS." In his experience, "There are still some medical people who, although aware of RLS, consider the disease psychological. . . . Centuries of prejudice tell doctors that what cannot be seen is in the mind."

WHY NO ONE SEEMS TO KNOW ABOUT RLS

RLS is largely unknown to the general public and, despite much scientific progress in recent decades, also eludes many in the medical profession. The neurologists and sleep experts I interviewed gave medical schools a failing grade. Take as an example the training of neurologist Dr. William Ondo:

> I graduated in 1991. I never heard of RLS in med school, never heard of it in internship, and barely heard of it in my neurology residency. I knew then that there was something called RLS. I thought the only treatment was Klonopin. My residency program had a well-known sleep center; however, 90 percent of what you learn is sleep apnea, then narcolepsy, and that's about it.

The subject of sleep has been overlooked by most medical schools—an astonishing oversight given that humans spend a third of their lives asleep, and that so many lives are brutally disordered by sleep deprivation. That omission is being remedied, but even so, RLS appears in the curricula only rarely. The result has been an entire medical community that is largely ignorant of the disease. Indeed, the 2003 Sleep in America poll conducted by the National Sleep Foundation found that only 3 percent of those reporting RLS symptoms had their disease diagnosed by a physician.[2]

A powerful indictment was made in a 1998 report delivered to Congress from the National Commission on Sleep Disorders Research by Dr. William C. Dement, world-renowned sleep expert: "The diagnosis and treatment of sleep disorders in primary care medicine today is essentially zero."[3] The tough report included RLS in the "epidemic of more than 40 million undiagnosed and untreated, or misdiagnosed and mistreated, chronically ill sleep disorders victims."[4] This epidemic was found to be a cause of "family dysfunction, workplace accidents, automobile crashes, lost education and income opportunities, disability, and premature death."[5]

All sleep disorders get shortchanged by most doctors. Many experts I interviewed agreed with Dr. Dement's contention that "the practice of medicine ends when the patient falls asleep." Dr. Dement added, "All our studies add up to about five thousand patients whose records have been painstakingly scrutinized. *In this mass of medical records we have yet to discover even one specific sleep disorder diagnosis. . . .* We are talking of around fifty thousand patient years without a single sleep disorder being recognized."[6]

Dr. Dement referred to polls showing that 49 percent of all adults suffer from insomnia and 12 percent have trouble sleeping *every night.* "Surveys eliciting the characteristic symptomology of restless legs syndrome have suggested a prevalence of 15 percent of all adults."[7] "The worst problem," according to Dr. Dement, "is the lack of medical school education. How can we expect primary care physicians to recognize the many victims of sleep disorders in their practice if physicians failed to diagnose, or even identify, one in three adults who suffer from insomnia?"[8]

Lack of awareness is also a problem in other countries. Dr. Pasquale Montagna has written that despite the efforts of his colleagues to inform the Italian public and fellow doctors, "In all my professional life of twenty-four years I have had only one patient referred to me for RLS by a primary care physician." Ironically, Dr. Montagna's fellow neurologists at Bologna were among the pioneers in RLS and PLM research.

The problem isn't new. "I am a retired general surgeon," wrote John M. Hoffer, of Oxford, Connecticut, whose mother had RLS "which was never diagnosed properly and which she aptly called 'the jitters.' I never learned anything about the syndrome in medical school and only saw a reference to it in a short article in one of the medical 'throw-away' journals."

Only recently did the Food and Drug Administration approve a drug specifically for use by RLS patients. On May 5, 2005, the

The late Dr. Richard L. Levin, former RLS Foundation board member and distinguished pathologist, analyzed the status of RLS in the medical community:

> There are many reasons why RLS and PLM have been in the background of medical knowledge, but the primary problem is that they aren't accepted as true entities by the medical community.
>
> Aside from the typical PLM twitches seen on polysomnographic studies, there are no concrete ways to make RLS or PLM diagnoses. Doctors must rely on victims' descriptions of weird feelings in the legs that are relieved by motor activity. And those feelings are being recounted, typically, by stressed-out, sleep-deprived patients who are too easily categorized as neurotics.
>
> The specialty of sleep medicine is populated by pulmonologists and neurologists. The pulmonologists are more interested in sleep apnea and narcolepsy than in RLS, a neurologic disease. The neurologists, however, are up against a catch-22: they are more likely to be interested in, and informed about, RLS than the pulmonologists, but they are dependent on referrals from general practitioners, who are too often unaware of the disease.
>
> Reviewing standard medical textbooks of internal medicine recently, I found no changes, or only minimal changes, in their coverage of RLS or PLM. The subject was not broached in my medical training in the '50s.
>
> With notable exceptions, there has been little coverage of RLS in the popular medical journals. There has been increased coverage recently in the specialty journals—articles by a cadre of familiar researchers in what amounts to "preaching to the choir."
>
> Another problem is the absence of reliable, nontoxic therapy for RLS. Physicians are hesitant to enter areas that are still experimental and where there have been standards of practice only since 1999.
>
> Finally, there are too many MDs who are derelict about staying current and availing themselves of the new concepts of medicine in spite of continuing medical education requirements.

drug ropinirole (Requip) was approved for RLS. Like other RLS medications likely to get approval in the near future, ropinirole is a dopamine agonist that substitutes for dopamine in the nervous system. Previously, some drugs used to treat other conditions were prescribed for RLS and were helpful. Hence, for RLS medications, there have been no advertisements of the sort that have become such an intimate part of our lives. This situation, happily, will continue to change since pharmaceutical companies are actively conducting studies on several different medications for RLS.

Perhaps another reason many people don't know about RLS is that *restless legs syndrome* is an unfortunate name that makes the disease sound trivial and easy to ignore. We have already noted that doctors often fail to ask their patients about sleep, but patients need to bear some responsibility for not bringing up the subject of their sleep. In fact, according to a 1995 Gallup poll, nearly 70 percent of people who have difficulty sleeping don't discuss sleep problems with their doctor at all.[9] Perhaps it's not surprising that people may be reluctant to talk about an affliction with such a trivial-sounding name and such hard-to-describe symptoms.

One of the greatest barriers to identifying RLS is the victims' fear that they won't be taken seriously. There is good reason for such fear, but as Dr. Robert Pascualy, of the Providence Hospital Sleep Disorders Center in Seattle, has pointed out, that reluctance may result in "maladaptive patterns," such as relying on alcohol to induce sleep—patterns that make patients' general health, and the disease itself, worse.

Thanks to the work of the RLS Foundation and pioneering doctors, the odds are changing in favor of nightwalkers. Your chances of knowing what you have, or of a doctor's knowing what you have—and of his or her knowing what to do about it—are improving. We need progress to be more rapid, especially given the amount of avoidable anguish in our nation's bedrooms, but there is more good news than bad. The RLS Foundation now receives more letters like this one, from a woman in Maryland: "After years of inquiries, I have found a doctor who prescribed something which relieves my RLS. It seems like a miracle to sleep all night!"

Asked in a January 2006 interview whether the last few years had seen a significant increase in sleep and RLS studies in medical schools, Dr. Richard Allen, a pioneer in RLS research, replied, "There has been progress, but not much, and certainly not enough. Only a few universities provide the kind of courses that meet our needs." A more hopeful view was presented by a colleague who said, "There is still real lack of teaching on the subject of sleep, including RLS. However, there is a reason for optimism. In the last few years the American Institute of Medicine has come up with standards for medical schools. And in association with that, the number of sleep centers has boomed, so I can't imagine there's a medical school that doesn't have some affiliation with a sleep center. As for RLS, now that there's an approved drug, Requip, it makes a big difference."

WHEN DOCTORS AND NURSES GET RLS

If it is frustrating for patients to be told by doctors that RLS is a sign of a psychological disorder, think how frustrating it is for some doctors to discover that they themselves have a disease that they failed to diagnose and treat. Many people are disheartened for years, sometimes decades, in their efforts to find out what plagues them at night. But are medical professionals more easily able to obtain an accurate diagnosis and sound advice? Not always.

Dr. Frankie Roman suffered from RLS during his entire medical training.

> I remember many a long night on call, I paced the hospital hallways trying to relieve the burning and aching in my legs.
>
> Occasionally, I evaluated patients who described my own symptoms. I would reassure the patient that he/she "had nothing" and if absolutely necessary prescribe a quinine-based drug for the vague and all-encompassing diagnosis of leg cramps. Then I would instruct the nurses not to page me for such a trivial problem and rush back to the house officer's call room to deal with my own restless legs and overall fatigue. Many a day I missed morning report, unable to wake up on time. And on days when I did make it, I would be confused, irritable, and fatigued.

It was only when Dr. Roman became a fellow in sleep disorders medicine at Scripps Clinic and Research Foundation that he discovered what had tormented him for so many years. "In my defense, albeit a poor one, I had absolutely no exposure to sleep disorders during college, medical school, or residency." Citing a survey of U.S. medical schools, Dr. Roman observed that less than two hours of teaching time is devoted to sleep topics.[10] In thirty-seven schools the subject was ignored altogether. It's no wonder that so many cases of RLS are misdiagnosed or undiagnosed.

Laura Schmidt, of Garland, Texas, a registered nurse, was for years unable to find help or even a diagnosis for her restless legs syndrome.

> I could not find anything in my research to help. . . . In my late thirties I started seeing doctors because I was falling asleep while

driving. . . . I tried meditation, self-hypnosis, wine at bedtime, warm milk, hot baths, relaxation tapes, getting drunk, herbs, vitamins—any suggestion made I tried. But still I would watch the sun set and the sun rise.

When I told doctors this, they said, "You were up *all* night?" and you could hear the doubt in their voice. I was told I was depressed, anxious, stressed, and many medications were given to no avail. . . . For years I was passed from doctor to doctor. The consensus was that nothing was physically wrong.

Then I had a sleep study which showed all this muscle movement (the technician in the morning said, "Lord, you must be exhausted, your legs moved all night long"). I tried medication after medication. Some helped for a night or two and then nothing. I still had no name for my problem. More research! Nothing! New doctor! New tests! I had a muscle and nerve biopsy—nonspecific morphological changes. EMG—disturbances consistent with nothing etc.! etc.! New doctor—sleep-deprived EEG—nothing! Medication after medication without much relief. And still no name.

As the years passed, Ms. Schmidt became too exhausted, anemic, and malnourished to care for others; she had to take a leave from nursing. But her persistence paid off. Eventually she found a neurologist who diagnosed RLS with nocturnal myoclonus. She discovered the RLS Foundation and contacted other people with RLS in her area. "The first time I talked to other people who had similar problems was like catching a lifeline thrown to a drowning person. Since then, thanks to the foundation, I have talked to many people who also have RLS and fight it on a daily basis." With the help of a sleep specialist, with medication, and with the support of her family, she was able to regain control of her life.

Edith C. Tuomala, of Cleveland, Ohio, was a registered nurse who began consulting doctors about her RLS in 1937. "No one knew anything and just pooh-poohed it as a figment of my imagination."

Another registered nurse, Sydney Jean Smith, of Kathleen, Florida, came from a family in which her father, mother, and daughter all suffered sensorimotor restlessness. The stress and long hours of her medical field made her own symptoms that much more dangerous.

The hospital wanted me to change to the 3:00 p.m. to 11:00 p.m. shift. I was still getting enough sleep to live a normal active life, but I noticed that after work I had to walk before I was able to get to sleep.

I transferred to operating room staff, and on one occasion went to work after a bad night of walking and only two hours of sleep. Driving home after working thirteen hours, I went to sleep and woke up on the wrong side of the road with a semi truck facing me. Having survived that, I knew it was time to see a doctor, but I had no idea what kind of doctor.

A few days later we had an eighty-three-year-old female patient who was awake every two hours and could only find relief by walking. Her doctor told me she had restless legs syndrome. He also told me to see a neurologist, which I did.

In an interview with the author, the pathologist Dr. Richard Levin reported experiencing RLS in varying degrees of intensity for thirty-five years. As his experience shows, even physicians can find their sensorimotor symptoms misattributed to psychiatric problems.

While I was in psychotherapy for anxiety at the time of my divorce in 1979, a therapist, a Freudian MD, spent about five sessions having me relate data about the relationship of which leg became initially involved, the identity of the person I was with at the time, and the geographical position of that person.

For instance, if symptoms began while sitting in a movie, [he asked] which leg was initially involved, who was I with (usually a female), and what was her position next to me—on the right or left side? Then we repeated the whole exercise for when symptoms began at dinner, at a concert, playing bridge, etc.

It is now painfully obvious, from the point of time, money, and what effect his implications had on the future of each relationship, that he did not have a clue as to what was really going on. When the left leg correlated with a person sitting at my left, this was felt to represent hidden anger. If on the right, he didn't have an obvious explanation. He screwed my head around to the point where I didn't know how I really felt about anybody or anything. He also succeeded in convincing me that my RLS symptoms were psychosomatic.

At this time I was forty-seven years old and knew that something was wrong with my nervous system but couldn't put a name on it. Luckily, at that time the RLS was in its early stages and fairly easily dealt with by taking hot showers and massaging my legs when necessary.

RLS really took hold in 1991 when my convalescence after coronary bypass was made especially miserable by my having to walk at home for hours at night before I could get some sleep by becoming exhausted. My chest incisions were not ready for such activity and kept me informed about their unhappiness.

My nonpsychiatric colleagues were also of little help, with varying degrees of disbelief and suggestions that I should seek psychotherapy. My ex-wife used to get on my back by stating that my need to move around at night was really hidden hostility toward her.

Dr. Levin finally diagnosed himself with RLS in 1991 and was started on Sinemet, which relieved his symptoms. As Dr. Levin concluded, "Now if we can only educate the medical profession as to diagnosis and therapy, then life will really feel rewarding."

It seems that the medical status of doctors and nurses has done little over the years to elevate them above fellow victims in their quest for relief. In the past, even doctors and nurses who knew what they had often didn't know what to do about it. And still today recognition may come slowly. Even after a correct diagnosis, managing medications and coping with side effects pose new challenges. But fortunately the medical community is becoming more aware of restless legs syndrome, and we can now expect to see accelerating progress toward rapid diagnosis, effective treatment, and someday a cure.

CHAPTER 3

Do I Have RLS?

*The red shoes had grown fast to her feet, and so dance she did,
and dance she must, over field and meadow, in rain and sunshine,
by day and by night. It was most horrible at night.*

—HANS CHRISTIAN ANDERSEN, "THE RED SHOES"

The odds of your getting RLS are determined by your sex (more women get it than men), genes (it's familial in about 50 percent of cases), age (older persons are more vulnerable), and by acquired conditions that can trigger the affliction (an iron deficiency, for example). People with RLS may have mild symptoms for many years, but the condition is often progressive, worsening with age.

How can a disease as widespread and debilitating as RLS remain largely unknown and untreated, especially in an era noted for so many major medical discoveries? In addition to ignorance, part of the problem is the nature of the disease. Restless legs *syndrome* involves a complex of symptoms that cannot simply be confirmed by a laboratory test. Further, diagnosis is complicated by the variety of possible causes. About half of cases are familial, others are either idiopathic (cause unknown) or related to other medical conditions like kidney disease or iron deficiency.

How do you and your doctor decide whether you have RLS?

Only in recent years have diagnostic standards been clarified. To assess whether your condition is indeed RLS, your doctor will begin by ascertaining whether you have the four essential criteria outlined below.

THE FOUR ESSENTIAL CRITERIA

A four-point description of RLS symptoms was developed by the International RLS Study Group (IRLSSG), which was formed in 1993 with the substantial aid of physicians. It now includes over 140 doctors from more than two dozen countries.

By May 1994, the IRLSSG was able to hold the first international symposium on RLS—an event that inspired an era of close cooperation among RLS researchers in several countries; in RLS research, as in other fields, medical pioneers in the United States are increasingly involved with, and indebted to, their colleagues in other nations.

In May 2002 the original diagnostic criteria were updated at an international diagnostic workshop at the National Institutes of Health in Washington, D.C.; the new criteria have been approved by the IRLSSG.[1] Thus, a physician making a diagnosis would strongly suspect RLS if a patient experienced:

1. An irritating need, urge, or even compulsion to move the legs—and, in more severe cases, arms—that can be highly distressing. This urge is usually associated with unpleasant abnormal sensations, such as burning, crawling, prickling, or jolting feelings.
2. Symptoms that are worse, or exclusively present, when the patient is at rest, sitting for a prolonged period or lying down.
3. Symptoms that can be relieved by activity as long as it is contin-

ued. The most common activity is walking, but stretching, shaking, massaging, or striking the legs can help. Mental activity and arousal also reduce symptoms.

4. Sensations that are worse in the evening or during the night. Such timing suggests that, as with asthma and some other diseases, the body's internal clock, which sets the circadian rhythm, plays a role.

While reviewing these criteria with your doctor, you will likely determine whether you have RLS and whether your case is mild, moderate, or severe. Mild cases are intermittent, whereas severe cases are daily and persistent. The most severe cases are referred to as *refractory*, which means they are obstinate and unresponsive to treatment. If moderately afflicted, one must walk occasionally. If very severely afflicted, one must walk for hours—sometimes from dusk till dawn, as I did night after night for more than five years. It's impossible for people who don't have the affliction to understand, but informed neurologists and medical dictionaries agree: its victims *must* move to obtain relief.

THE ASSOCIATION WITH PLM

As though the tribulations of RLS weren't enough, at least 80 percent of people with RLS also have an affliction called *periodic limb movements* (PLM), twitches that occur every twenty to forty seconds.

These jerks were initially called *nocturnal myoclonus* by the English neurologist Sir Charles Putnam Symonds in 1953. Their association with RLS was uncovered by a group of Italian neurologists in the early 1960s.[2] The prevalence of PLM, like RLS—and, alas, so many other ailments—usually worsens with age.

Periodic limb movements cause leg jerks or kicks during non-dreaming (or nonREM) sleep. These movements may be harder on bed partners than on the victims, since the afflicted often don't realize they are twitching and complain only of vague symptoms such as irritability and feeling tired. It is not uncommon for the awakened, and understandably irritated, partner to complain about being kicked before the victim is aware of the movements. One doctor reported bruises on a victim's legs—the result of the bed partner kicking back.

Treatments for PLM and RLS are almost always the same, so I won't include PLM each time RLS is mentioned. (For an excellent source on PLM, see papers by Dr. Sonia Ancoli-Israel, professor of psychiatry at the University of California in San Diego, who has devoted many years to research on PLM.)

Periodic limb movements shouldn't be confused with the full-body jolts (called *hypnic jerks*) experienced on the edge of sleep by virtually everyone at one time or another. Nor should RLS be confused with painful nighttime leg cramps, which are usually treated with quinine.

Like RLS, PLM in its severe form can kill sleep. You've heard it, or said it, many times: "I didn't sleep a wink last night," or "I doubt that I slept two hours." What that usually means, according to sleep experts, is that the person slept fitfully, was subject to frequent awakenings, and got up feeling fatigued. But discomfort tricked their memories: they did sleep, and the odds are that they slept several hours. Periodic limb movements don't usually kill sleep for hours at a time. It leaves that terrible task to RLS.

OTHER ASSOCIATED FEATURES

While RLS may, in many cases, be a familial condition, it has also been associated with a number of other disorders. They are *associated with* but not necessarily *a cause of* RLS.

Although it is hard to define these conditions with precision, they fall roughly into three categories:

First, there are disorders that are known or suspected to cause RLS. The most important include iron-deficiency anemia, pregnancy (usually in the third trimester), and kidney failure (end-stage renal disease). Other factors include peripheral neuropathy, fibromyalgia, surgery or certain other physical traumas, lumbar radiculopathy, rheumatoid arthritis, and the use of most antidepressant and antipsychotic medications. Deficiencies of magnesium, folate, and vitamin B_{12} have also been associated, anecdotally, with RLS. The evidence for the relationship between RLS and these conditions varies, with some connections being clearer than others. Venous insufficiency is occasionally mentioned but does not have much research support.

Second, there are other conditions confused with or commonly occurring with RLS, but the degree of causality is even less evident, such as attention-deficit/hyperactivity disorder (ADHD). It is recommended that your child be examined for RLS if he or she has the following symptoms: difficulty falling asleep, difficulty staying asleep, signs of sleep deprivation such as irritability and restlessness (during day or night). Some researchers also put fibromyalgia and diabetes in this category—the category in which evidence of a causal relation is weaker or more indirect, and in which both RLS and these conditions may have a common cause. For example, diabetes often causes peripheral neuropathy, which may result in RLS.

Finally, there are conditions, like fatigue or depression, which may aggravate or be caused by RLS.

ONSET: EARLY VERSUS LATE

For many, RLS is a lifelong affliction. Since RLS and PLM can begin in childhood, many victims have suffered for decades. Recent research shows that what has been called "growing pains" can be early-stage RLS. No one has conducted more studies of RLS/PLM in children than Dr. Daniel Picchietti, whose teenage son, Matt, spoke to patients and doctors at the first national conference of the RLS Foundation on September 27, 2002. So far, little is known about the special problems posed in the identification and treatment of juvenile RLS. It is a hopeful sign that the talks of both father and son were heavily attended.

"Kids are not little adults," Dr. Picchietti reminded the audience after his son described what it was like to suffer with RLS in elementary and high school. "The diagnosis is more difficult than with adults," the father reported. "Symptoms are typically mild and intermittent. It's important to get a family history because the parents may have RLS. A sleep study may also be a good idea." The treatment is complex, Dr. Picchietti said, and always involves a rigid sleep schedule that is consistent and appropriate for age, avoidance of almost all caffeine, supplementary iron if it's deficient, and perhaps, under a doctor's supervision, medication.

A fortunate few children and adults experience remissions, which can last for months or years. No one yet knows why these welcome respites appear or disappear.

In the early stages of the disease (whether early or late onset), sleep is less affected, especially among the lucky people who go to sleep fast and sleep soundly. Legs will be moving, perhaps from both RLS and PLM, but at that stage only the bed partner may notice. Victims eventually become aware of a need not only to stretch their legs but also to stretch them over and over, to move them around, to get up and walk. That may not be easily accomplished, as many agitated airline passengers, restrained by food and drink carts and seat belt signs, have testified.

For many nightwalkers the subversive villain is scarcely noticeable at the beginning. RLS creeps in, at first imperceptibly. These late-onset nightwalkers are often first conscious of discomfort while having to lie still for a prolonged period, perhaps as a result of some other disease or a surgical procedure.

THE AGE FACTOR

One of the ironies of age is that, just when we need them most, we often become less able to perform the very functions that would improve our health or keep disease from getting worse. For example, I now have severe degenerative disease of the lower spine (osteoarthritis) that makes walking painful. What would I have done a few years ago when RLS forced me to walk for hours every night? And before a new medication reduced the RLS?

In his amusing book *Making It Through Middle Age*, William Attwood wrote of the aging body: "If it works, it hurts; if it doesn't hurt it isn't working."[3] Indeed, there's enough going wrong in those troubled years without adding the indignity, discomfort, and sometimes agony of legs that insist on being moved for hours every night. "What happens then?" asks Mary V. Rodenbarger, of Niles, Michigan.

My mother is seventy-four and has many health problems. She is not able to walk too well at any time, so "walking it off" in the middle of the night has become a real challenge for her. I am fifty-two years old and have emphysema. It is of real concern to me that the day will come when I simply cannot walk around. What happens then? Have PLM and RLS symptoms ever driven someone completely bonkers? My symptoms first began during my late teen years. Currently I experience problems every day and night sometimes to the point that even my arms begin to feel crawly. I recently told my husband that maybe when I die, he could find someone to give my body to for research.

A leading neurologist did her best to help a ninety-two-year-old patient who had severe RLS and was debilitated with arthritis. "Can you imagine it?" the neurologist asked. "She can't get up and walk because of the arthritis, but she can't sit still because of the RLS. Recently, she needed an angiogram but couldn't tolerate being strapped down for the procedure." During an angiogram, patients are immobilized while a catheter is slowly eased from the groin through the main artery to the heart. I've heard of two cases in which patients, despite restraints, had to move, tried to do so, and fouled up the examination. One of them, a patient in a Milwaukee hospital, died.

The neurologist's patient, like many of the elderly, suffered side effects from larger doses of medications. "We had to keep making adjustments," the neurologist said. "With the elderly, combining two or three lower doses of different drugs is usually more effective than large doses of a single medication."

GENDER

Restless legs syndrome is more prevalent in women than men. Women, in fact, increase their risk for RLS with the number of children they bear. A recent German study involving over four thousand individuals concluded that "women with no children had similar prevalence to men, while women with three or more children had more than three times the risk of having RLS."[4] This finding is corroborated by another recent study in which significantly more women reported early-onset RLS compared to men.[5]

It may be that iron and hormones play critical roles, particularly since so many women not only often experience RLS for the first time during pregnancy, but also find that their symptoms often disappear after delivery, especially if they haven't been nightwalkers before.

WHAT TO DO IF YOU HAVE RLS

First, find a doctor who is either familiar with RLS or interested in learning. An excellent starting point is Appendix D, the Health Care Providers directory in the back of this book. In addition, the RLS Foundation website, www.rls.org, maintains a directory of health care providers in your area that is updated frequently. Fellow sufferers in support groups are listed in Appendix B: Support Groups. The RLS website also offers a free "Online Community" with a "Forum for Discussion." You may want to look for a sleep disorder clinic in your area.

Next, urge your doctor to read the treatment algorithm for RLS. You can access this by going to www.mayo.edu/proceedings, clicking on July 2004, and then on the title "An Algorithm for the Management of Restless Legs Syndrome." Because there is no one remedy for restless legs syndrome, an informed doctor will assist you in the management of this disease. Effective treatment involves trial and error. What works for some will not work for others. Further, what works for you may do so only for a certain period. You and you doctor will want to work together to determine your best course of action.

In addition to the strategies developed with your doctor, there are options set out in Chapter 4 to help you sleep. Chapter 5 examines the medical therapies available.

Education is key. Your RLS may be familial, so explain the disease to relatives. It's possible that they share your nighttime woes and are as mystified as you may have been. Many letters from RLS patients describe families that have become dysfunctional. Irritable RLS victims, battered by fatigue, didn't know what they had or, even if they knew, were too proud to ask for help. Every family member suffered. Learning as much as you can about restless legs syndrome and sharing that knowledge with others can help you avoid those pitfalls.

As you learn about this serious illness, spread the word, even beyond your family. Inform others in and out of medical fields. Arm yourself with pamphlets from the RLS Foundation, and share the information freely. Public awareness is the first step to relieving suffering and finding a cure.

WHAT'S IN A NAME?

Robert Balkam, a former salesman and former RLS Foundation board member, once remarked, "If restless legs syndrome were a product, I'd have a terrible time selling it. With that name no one would take it seriously."

If you think you may have RLS, don't be put off by the name. *Restless legs syndrome* is a lousy name for a serious disease. It gives no hint of how devastating the affliction can be. Although a cause of misery for millions, RLS is hard to describe and diagnose. Even in the unlikely event that people with its symptoms have heard of RLS, they may be unwilling to complain to their doctors about something that sounds so odd and easy to dismiss.

There you are, fatigued, hollow-eyed, irritable, and possibly depressed from having to ambulate night after night, and someone asks you, "What's the problem?"

"I have restless legs," you reply. "Can't sleep."

In most cases you might as well have said that you had the vapors.

"That's too bad" is a typical response. "Have you tried sleeping pills?"

You are tempted to snarl, "Of course I've tried sleeping pills. I've also tried aspirin, ibuprofen, muscle relaxants, tranquilizers, antidepressants, vitamins, mineral supplements, quinine, allergy drugs, hot soaks, cold soaks, exercises, diets, acupuncture, astrological consultations, and a dozen doctors."

But you don't snarl, out of fear that your testiness will only be interpreted as a sign of a mental disorder. It's bad enough to have relatives and friends think that your problem is psychological. "A few sessions on a psychiatrist's couch would solve it," Aunt Sophie says to her weary husband. "Restless legs! It's his head that's restless."

Those of us who have staggered around a bedroom instead of sleeping are understandably resentful of people who sleep eight hours each night. And that resentment grows whenever we see in someone's eyes a suspicion that our problem is neurotic rather than neurological.

How much worse, then, to encounter such suspicion in a doctor or nurse, an amazing number of whom haven't heard of restless legs. Many others, who *have* heard the name, shrug and change the subject. Although people with the severest form of RLS can lose jobs, alienate friends and family, have accidents caused by sleep deprivation, and even consider killing themselves, doctors and nurses, like the rest of us, are likely to feel that if it doesn't *sound* serious, it probably isn't. (A woman in Georgia wrote to medical columnist Dr. Peter Gott, stating that she had been diagnosed with "reckless legs" and urging him to please write on the subject.)

One's first thought on hearing "restless legs" is perhaps of children in kindergarten, some of whom, recent research has shown, may actually have RLS, but most of whom are merely suffering from juvenile fidgetiness. Restless legs syndrome also sounds like a fad disease—one of those tough-to-test, ill-defined afflictions that are popularized in the tabloid press and then fade away.

But although the name lacks gravitas, the world's most distinguished neurologists and sleep disorder specialists take RLS very seriously. So why don't they change the name? Why, as a matter of fact, did they drop the eponymic *Ekbom's syndrome*, which does have weight and was named after the Swedish neurologist who conducted studies of the affliction in the 1940s?

It may be because the revered Swede himself coined the term *restless legs*, though he probably wouldn't have objected if the medical community had decided to honor him by sticking to *Ekbom's syndrome*. He might better have called it *asthenia crurum paraesthetica* ("irritable legs") or *focal quiescoegenic nocturnal akathisia*, or even *anxietas tibiarum*, as RLS was inexactly called in the nineteenth century. Consider the afflictions listed by the National Organization for Rare Disorders, of which there are nearly a thousand: Primary agammaglobulinemias? Erythrokeratodermia progressive symmetrical ichthyosis? Almost any of them sound more consequential than restless legs syndrome.

Those who oppose a change point out that RLS *is* close to the ideal descriptive term for the sensation. To greater effect, they argue that so many scientific papers have been written on the subject within the last few years that RLS is now firmly embedded in medical literature.

The best argument I've seen for the status quo came from Canadian David Shaler, who maintained a helpful and busy website devoted to RLS in the 1990s. Shaler outlined these disadvantages of using the term:

> Ekbom's syndrome has three disadvantages. First, it is used in the psychiatric literature for a delusional condition in which someone actually believes there are insects crawling under the skin, rather than just having a sensation of insects crawling under the skin. Second, it provides no information about the nature of the condition. Third, the use of names for diseases is disfavored currently in the medical field. What usually works is a descriptive phrase that can be turned into an easily remembered acronym, such as AIDS.

Shaler also pointed out the benefit of the label "restless legs." Not only is it a "catchy" term, whose abbreviation, RLS, is unusual and easy to remember, but also a change of name would cause confusion and result in lost access to information.

But despite these arguments for the status quo, passionate protests are made by those favoring *Ekbom's syndrome* (or *disorder* or *disease*). A particularly trenchant argument for change was made in a letter to the author in 2000 by Dr. Charlotte McCutchen, when she was program director of Sleep Disorders Medicine at the National Institute of Neurological Disorders and Stroke (NINDS):

> If we called a disease such as Parkinsonism "shaking head syndrome" we would get the same reaction from the public, Congress, and grant reviewers that we get now for "restless legs syndrome." When I was in training, RLS was taught to me as "Ekbom's syndrome," which, like Parkinson's, Alzheimer's, and Huntington's, is a name that may be obscure but doesn't generate laughter, or a mental block against taking it seriously.
>
> The name "restless legs syndrome" is a definite liability for this disease, and I have seen the name do everything from result in an unfundable score on a grant application to incredulous comments from congressmen, who want to know "What's next, a demand for funding for 'ingrown toenail syndrome'?"
>
> Yet when I have brought this up at professional meetings, I get surprised glares, as though I were stepping on hallowed ground. The problem the field doesn't see is that when you are fighting to the death for the appreciation of the seriousness of a disease, you shoot yourself and the disease in the foot by referring to it with a title laypeople find ridiculous, no matter how accurately descriptive it may be. And no matter how comfortable people who are familiar with the disease may be with this ridiculous moniker, the fact is they are turning off the very people we need so desperately to reach with our message—those people who *don't* have a familiarity with it.
>
> And the argument that the descriptive term should be kept because it is accurate cuts no ice with me either. It is not *just* restless legs. The sensory system, the dopamine system, and the opiate system, to name a few, are all involved. The patient is systemically affected, with disrupted sleep and daytime function. To name it after just one of its aspects is inaccurate.

There have been numerous name changes in medicine. Elephant-man syndrome was referred to as von Recklinghausens disease but more recently is usually referred to as neurofibromatosis. Leprosy is now referred to as Hansen's disease, general paresis of the insane is now called neurosyphilis, mongolism is now Down syndrome.

I wish the RLS folks could do the same, instead of tilting against an unnecessary windmill. The very real problems they face are challenge enough.

In Europe, *Ekbom syndrome* is widely employed, but in most countries the English term, or a translation of it, is used. The phrase *restless legs* sounds just as trivial and frivolous when translated into another tongue or, as sometimes happens, when mixed with another language. (In German, for example, the chief support group is known as Deutsche Restless Legs Vereinigung.)

According to neurologist Pasquale Montagna, *restless legs* is an impediment to wider interest in and treatment of the disease in Italy. " 'Restless legs' does not sound like a thing of serious concern," he wrote. "Some people laugh at me when I mention this term, and I have to emphasize the problem. 'Ekbom disease' would sound more professional."

Letters from nightwalkers also reflect a similar dissatisfaction. John D. Lee wrote to Shaler's website that "the seriousness of the problem gets minimized and denigrated by such a goofy name. . . . Unfortunately, the current name invites derision, especially by the uneducated." To which Marilyn Helleberg added, "I even hesitate to talk to people about my problem because it does sound so psychosomatic."

Those who favored calling it Ekbom's syndrome, always a minority, are heard from less and less frequently. American medical journals, where any continuing battle would be waged, don't use that name at all.

One thing is certain: restless legs does make it easier for people to ridicule the disease, but their numbers will dwindle as public awareness grows. If you suffer the symptoms of RLS, you know how serious they are. With persistence you can find other people—fellow nightwalkers and medical providers—who will understand as well.

CHAPTER 4

Sleep and How to Get More of It

If sleep does not serve an absolutely vital function, then it is the biggest mistake the evolutionary process has ever made.

—ALLAN RECHTSCHAFFEN, DIRECTOR OF THE UNIVERSITY OF CHICAGO SLEEP LABORATORY, *SMITHSONIAN*, NOVEMBER 1978

Without food, rats die in 16 days; without sleep, 17 days.

—*U.S. NEWS & WORLD REPORT*, AUGUST 18, 1997

Now blessings light on him that first invented this same sleep! It covers a man all over, thoughts and all, like a cloak; 'tis meat for the hungry, drink for the thirsty, heat for the cold, and cold for the hot. 'Tis the current coin that purchases all the pleasures of the world cheap; and the balance that sets the king and the shepherd, the fool and the wise man even.

—MIGUEL DE CERVANTES, *DON QUIXOTE DE LA MANCHA*

Restless legs syndrome is not normally thought of as a life-threatening disease. The creepy-crawly sensations, while painful and distressing, do not seem to signal any lasting damage to the body. After decades of symptoms, nightwalkers are still walking around.

But that's the problem: we're walking around instead of sleeping. Sleep deprivation can pose an enormous danger to anyone, and people with RLS are more likely than most to suffer severe, long-term sleep loss. For most nightwalkers, the single biggest challenge we face is to get enough sleep.

As only the pauper can fully appreciate wealth, as only the ill can fully rejoice in health, so only the sleep-deprived can fully enjoy sleep. When even the hope for repose is gone, banished by the feeling that rest has been lost forever, then one begins to yearn for eternal sleep.

In its most severe form, RLS forces victims to stay awake all night, as I often did. Bedtime for me became a dreaded time. I would lie down but within minutes that terrifying creepy-crawly feeling would compel me to get up and walk. In the "hours of the wolf"—the bleak depth of the night from about one o'clock to five—I thought a thousand times, "I can't stand this anymore." Sleep deprivation can cause not only intense physical fatigue but also mental collapse and despair.

At some level, it's not surprising to learn that everyone's tired and grumpy, and driving while sleepy. After all, it's common knowledge that we're all stressed out and doing too much. At another level, though, the statistics are truly alarming. For example, the National Institutes of Health estimate that 40 million Americans suffer from chronic sleep disorders, the vast majority of which, like RLS and PLM, remain *undiagnosed and untreated*, and yet another 20 to 30 million people suffer intermittent sleep-related problems.[1] Let's face it, as a nation, we're pooped.

Despite the lack of sleep in the general population, though, few doctors pay attention to sleep at all, let alone the harm that can result from insufficient or disordered sleep. More than 70 percent of adults have never been asked about the quality of their sleep by a physician, and fewer than 20 percent have ever initiated a discussion.[2] Sleep researchers have linked many ailments to inadequate sleep, including high blood pressure, depression, cardiovascular disease, and even obesity. As sleep expert Stanley Coren so eloquently put it, "Lack of sleep makes people clumsy, unhappy, stupid, and dead."[3] Another expert, Dr. William C. Dement, says there is no doubt that disordered sleep is physically and psychologically harmful. Sleep is at least as important to our well-being as exercise and good diet. "If sleep is mismanaged," he said, "we may be risking our lives. We are not healthy unless our sleep is healthy."[4]

The size of the problem is evident in all studies. It's huge, and growing. The U.S. surgeon general, Richard H. Carmona, reports that untreated sleep disorders affect 70 million Americans and cost the nation $15 billion a year in health care expenses.[5]

Surveys conducted by the National Sleep Foundation (NSF) show that 75 percent of adults report having sleep problems a few nights a week or more. This continues an upward trend in the prevalence of sleep problems—from 62 percent who experienced a sleep problem a few nights a week or more in 1999 and 2000, to 69 percent in 2001, to 74 percent in 2002, and 75 percent in 2005. In addition, more than 40 percent of adults experienced daytime sleepiness severe enough to interfere with their daily activities at least a few days each month, with 20 percent reporting persistent sleepiness a few days a week or more.[6]

The large 2005 Sleep in America poll, commissioned by the NSF, found that respondents were getting an average of 6.8 hours of sleep on weeknights and 7 hours on weekends.[7] Over the past several years, there has been a downward trend in the proportion of respondents who report sleeping 8 or more hours a night on weekdays (from 38 percent in 2001, to 30 percent in 2002, and 26 percent in 2005). Three-quarters of respondents said they experienced at least one symptom of a sleep disorder a few nights a week. Those symptoms include difficulty falling asleep, waking up a lot during the night, waking up too early and not being able to go back to sleep, waking up feeling unrefreshed, snoring, pauses in breathing, and having bothersome feelings in the legs.

Some results of sleep deprivation are predictable. For example, respondents said that not getting enough sleep made them feel more irritable, more likely to lose their patience around children, and likely to get angry while driving. Equally unsurprising, adults living with children got less sleep than those without children.

Use of sleep medicine is also on the rise. Some studies have reported that as many as 15 percent of people said they had used either a prescription or over-the-counter drug for sleep.

Age matters. Restorative, slow wave deep sleep makes up 20 percent of our sleep at the age of twenty-five but a mere 5 percent at sixty.[8] As Dr. Sonia Ancoli-Israel puts it, "It's a myth that sleeping less is part of getting old. It's not the need for sleep that changes, it's our ability to sleep well."[9]

Certainly sleep plays a vital role in our well-being. Some assert it is *the* most important predictor for longevity. Citing sleep and mortality studies, including a gigantic one conducted by the American Cancer Society, Dr. Dement concluded that "there is plenty of compelling evidence supporting the argument that sleep is the most important predictor of how long you will live, perhaps more important than whether you smoke, exercise, or have high blood pressure or cholesterol."[10] A California Department of Health study published in *Sleep* showed that people who get less than the recommended amount of sleep have a 70 percent higher death rate than those who get adequate sleep.[11]

None of those life-span studies prove a *causal* relationship between longevity and amount of sleep, but as Dr. Dement observes, "the results are extremely suggestive." He suggests the immune system may hold the answer here, since "there seems to be an intriguing and mysterious connection between sleep and the maintenance of our bodies through immune function and cell repair."[12]

Researchers may choose to include victims of auto accidents when citing the effect of sleep disorders on death rates. Studies have shown that drowsy drivers cause an average of 70,000 injuries every year and 1,550 deaths.[13] The annual cost of motor vehicle accidents in the United States is $13 billion.

In the 2005 Sleep in America poll, 60 percent of respondents reported that they had driven a vehicle while feeling fatigued and often drowsy, and almost two of every ten said that they had dozed off while driving at some point within the past year.[14] More frightening, 80 percent of regional pilots reported that they occasionally snooze in the cockpit, which, among other things, is illegal. When one adds RLS, and the stress it generates, to the effects of sleep deprivation on the immune system, the results are equally intriguing. That connection is explored more fully in Chapter 8.

If too few doctors pay attention to sleep problems, there is no shortage of advice from book, magazine, and newspaper publishers. All this guidance can get confusing: one book contains seventy-five suggestions on ways to obtain better sleep.

Sleep routines and sleep needs vary. The sleep-aid recommendations below are of a general nature but are especially appropriate for people over age fifty, since the most severe cases of RLS are found in that age group. For a more detailed review, read the final chapter of Dr. Dement's excellent 1999 book, *The Promise of Sleep*.[15]

It is important, while reviewing the suggestions for improved sleep below, to keep in mind that a consistent positive routine (like getting up at the same time every morning, cutting back on caffeine and alcohol, and avoiding long naps) is the most effective sleep aid. To that end, many find bedtime rituals can be helpful—

things like meditation or writing in a journal, or enjoying a cup of herbal tea or a warm bath.

The following strategies should be taken, as Dr. Dement suggests, as options—rules that can be broken if circumstances dictate. If, for example, you are a business executive preparing an urgent report, or a student cramming for an exam, you may occasionally have to stay up late. But the more regular you can be in your habits, the better success you'll have.

Option 1. Be regular. Go to bed at the same time every night and get up at the same time every morning.

Given the relation between RLS and circadian rhythm, your legs will be grateful to the degree to which you can put your body's biological clock on a schedule. If you miss sleep during the week, try to make up for lost sleep on the weekend. (About 10 percent of college undergraduates say they sleep eight or more hours on weeknights, but the figure rises by more than 70 percent on weekends.)[16] *The Promise of Sleep* cites evidence showing it was safe to assume that people can avoid dangerously high sleep debt by adding a relatively small amount of sleep to their normal sleep schedule, and this has not been disproved as of this writing.

Option 2. Use the bedroom and bed only for sleep and sex. Ideally you should think of your bed as the most comfortable or enjoyable place in the world.

Option 3. If you fail to fall asleep within twenty minutes, go to another room, or at least to a nearby chair, and read. But nothing too stimulating. Sir Walter Scott is perfect. This kind of diversion, which can help you avoid thinking of the bed with anxiety, works best for people whose RLS is mild.

Option 4. Avoid substances that aggravate RLS.

A. It's the caffeine, stupid! Anyone who has trouble sleeping should avoid caffeinated drinks and chocolate. There is evidence that caffeine intensifies RLS in children and perhaps in some adults. For example, Dr. Daniel Picchietti discovered, in a study of the comorbidity of ADHD and RLS, that soft drinks containing caffeine may aggravate both afflictions in children. Caffeine can stay in your system for up to twenty hours. Remember that caffeine may be included in some over-the-counter pain and cold remedies. Chocolate and many weight-loss aids also contain caffeine. If you are taking more than the equivalent of one cup of coffee a day (about 100 mg caffeine), gradual tapering off is recommended to avoid the nasty effects of caffeine withdrawal.

B. Alcohol is another culprit. Drink alcoholic beverages only moderately with dinner and not at all afterward. Alcohol exacerbates RLS symptoms and too much alcohol can bring on a rebound effect that will sabotage sleep three or four hours after the drink is consumed.

C. Nicotine can also disrupt sleep and worsen symptoms. Avoid it altogether to preserve sleep—and your life.

Option 5. It can be easier for RLS victims to nap in the afternoon than to sleep at night. But the general rule applies: avoid naps beyond midafternoon, and don't nap for more than an hour.

Option 6. Eat your evening meal at least three hours before bedtime. Eat lightly, as nutritionists advise. A light snack may be a good idea *if* you feel hungry at bedtime. Hunger can wake you up. But remember, so can overeating at night.

Option 7. Exercise, but not within four hours of bedtime unless it's related to low-energy sex. Fitness can improve the quality and quantity of sleep and is generally beneficial for mind and body, but nighttime exercise, especially the strenuous aerobic sort, not only impairs sleep but also worsens RLS. This stricture, however, wouldn't include mild stretching of the sort that some nightwalkers find helpful.

Option 8. Don't put your alarm clock where you can see its face; it can make you anxious. (Some people awaken periodically, worrying that the alarm may fail them. They should buy a second clock or pay for a wake-up telephone service.)

Option 9. Most people sleep best in a dark and quiet bedroom. (Use an eye mask or earplugs if necessary.)

Option 10. Try to reduce stress. That's not easy, especially for those of us whose limbs test us nightly, but the benefits of stress reduction are manifold, especially in bed. This is particularly true for Americans, who, according to many experts, are the most stressed on the globe. Games and other forms of social interaction can also reduce stress and enhance sleep.

Option 11. Use prescription drug therapies sparingly. Anything you use for more than three months, whether prescription or over-the-counter, should be monitored by your doctor. (Also consult your doctor about antidepressants; many aggravate RLS symptoms.)

Experts agree: before resorting to sleeping pills, RLS victims should look at all the possible causes of insomnia. If you can treat the underlying disease with whatever drugs you and your doctor find effective, you may be able to avoid taking medication for the insomnia. If sleeping pills are used, make sure to choose the sort that don't lead to development of tolerance and rebound insomnia. Two such drugs that have passed double-blind, controlled tests are Ambien and Halcion. Short-acting drugs like Ambien, Halcion, and Sonata are less likely to cause debilitating daytime "hangovers." They also reduce the likelihood of late-night falls suffered by people en route to the bathroom while under the influence of a sedative.

It is especially important for the elderly to ask questions about the conditions that might be causing sleep problems. Patients should review with their doctor the dosage and timing of *all* medications. Do they have side effects? Are the above options being em-

SLEEP DISORDER CENTERS

The American Academy of Sleep Medicine (AASM), formerly known as the American Sleep Disorders Association (ASDA), accredits sleep disorders laboratories and centers. In 1978 only 3 such centers existed. By 2002 there were 543, and by 2005, 794.

Readers who suspect that they have RLS may benefit from a visit to a sleep disorder center. While it is true that sufferers of restless legs syndrome have not always found assistance at such centers, the AASM (see Appendix A) is committed to making sure that its members can recognize RLS and PLM. They are expected either to treat it or provide advice as to where it can be treated.

According to AASM accreditation committee standards, "The Center must offer a full range of diagnostic and therapeutic techniques including but not limited to sleep-disordered breathing, restless legs syndrome, periodic limb movement disorder, parasomnias, narcolepsy, behavioral treatment of insomnia, and therapy for circadian rhythm disorders." Further, centers applying for new accreditation, or for renewal of their accreditation, must demonstrate their ability "to provide diagnostic and therapeutic services for restless legs syndrome and periodic limb movement disorder."

But remember not all sleep labs or sleep centers are accredited. When considering seeking help from such a service, check to see that it is fully accredited by the American Academy of Sleep Medicine. If it is not, it is unlikely to have RLS expertise and may not be very helpful. For a list of accredited centers go to www.sleepcenters.org.

ployed? Has advice been sought from a general practitioner or, in the case of severe RLS, perhaps a sleep specialist or a neurologist?

The search for sleep is as old as humankind. So is the list of nostrums.[17] Any or all of the above options may help nightwalkers, but nothing will help as much as enlisting your doctor in a search for the best strategy for treating the disease.

CHAPTER 5

Medical Help

Prayer indeed is good, but while calling on the gods
a man should himself lend a hand.

—HIPPOCRATES, *REGIMEN*

Imagine that you have read an article about RLS and are convinced that you have the disease. Eager to find out more about treatment or a possible cure, you seek advice from your doctor, who may not know what you are talking about. You may have to show him the article in order to convince him that you are indeed among the afflicted. What, then, do the two of you do?

You look at the *Physicians' Desk Reference* and, unless it was published in late 2005 or more recently, you discover that there is no specific medicine identified as a treatment for RLS. Why? Because only recently have pharmaceutical companies begun to invest the research time and money needed to obtain approval from the Food and Drug Ad-

NOTE: DO NOT TAKE ANY MEDICATION MENTIONED IN THIS BOOK WITHOUT CONSULTING YOUR DOCTOR.

ministration (FDA) for an RLS-specific drug. The good news is that the pharmaceutical companies, now aware that there are millions of people living with RLS in the United States and abroad, are seeking FDA approval for several medications that can be prescribed and advertised as treatments for RLS.

Such approval, which requires a large investment in research, is necessary even if the company wants only to identify a drug that is already approved for treating another disease as also appropriate for treating RLS. GlaxoSmithKline completed that research in 2004 and has now obtained FDA approval and begun marketing for treatment of RLS its dopamine agonist Requip—initially developed as a therapy for Parkinson's. Other pharmaceutical companies are certain to follow, although recent applicants will gain approval only after a year or more of trials.

The dopamine agonist Requip is one of a class of drugs called *dopaminergic agents,* that is, drugs that affect the processing of the neurotransmitter dopamine. Other drugs of various types may be used for RLS therapy, but only "off label," which simply means a drug is used for a purpose other than the one that it was designed for. Most prescription drugs used for RLS fall into four categories:

dopaminergic agents
benzodiazepines
narcotics/opioids and other analgesics
anticonvulsants

How do you and your doctor decide which of these drugs is likely to be the most effective—or whether drugs are needed at all? Since RLS can result from a combination of factors, both genetic and environmental, a medical evaluation is necessary. It should include

1. Reviewing the four essential criteria for diagnosis outlined in Chapter 3.
2. Questions about proper nutrition and sleep habits. Occasionally symptoms are triggered by an iron deficiency and can be subdued with iron supplements. A more remote possibility is that symptoms result from a vitamin or mineral deficiency or from an excess of caffeine.
3. A neurologic examination with emphasis on spinal cord functioning and nerves in the limbs.
4. A vascular exam to rule out disorders of the veins and arteries.

Once vitamin/mineral deficiencies and neurological and vascular abnormalities have been ruled out, you and your doctor will look for a medication that will help. Alas, no single drug works for everyone. There is no consensus among researchers and practitioners on what should be tried first, or in what sequence. Two researchers who have been studying RLS and PLM may choose differently when deciding which drug, or combination of drugs, to employ with a given patient. Some people are helped by a drug that has little effect on another RLS patient. One person may suffer unacceptable side effects from a drug that has no negative effects on another. In an interview with the author, Dr. Picchietti observes "that responses to medication often run in families." Factors aggravating RLS—pain, sleep deprivation, alcohol and caffeine use, lack of exercise, other medications (particularly antinausea and motion-sickness drugs), and drug interactions—may influence the choice of medication.

Given so many variables, and given that the newest drugs, the dopamine agonists, haven't been used long enough to provide definitive profiles, it's no wonder that multiple approaches are used. As with much of medicine, the treatment of RLS is as much an art as a science.

THE DOPAMINE CONNECTION

Dopamine is a neurotransmitter "that has been shown to be a key modulator in an astonishing array of human behaviors. Get too much dopamine in the brain and you hear voices, hallucinate and wrestle with twisted thoughts. Get too little of it and you cannot move."[1] It can cause you to throw a ball—or throw a tantrum. This mighty molecule brings us pleasure and elation; it can also, by shortchanging us, bring misery and even death.

Dopamine, identified as a neurotransmitter in the late 1950s, is used by nerve cells to "talk" to each other. The *dopamine system* includes all the nerve cells in the brain and spinal cord that either produce or respond to dopamine.

The major site for making dopamine is the *substantia nigra* ("black substance," or SN), which has some 400,000 neurons—a minuscule fraction of the 100 billion cells in the human brain—and is located deep in the brain stem. The SN manufactures all the dopamine needed by other nerve cells. It is the gradual death of nigral neurons that depletes the supply of dopamine in Parkinson's victims. The long axons of those dopaminergic cells connect to many locations around the higher centers of the brain, where dopamine is released when electrical impulses move along the axons. The released dopamine can then influence the activity of its target cells, generally called *postsynaptic neurons* (meaning they are on the receiving side of the connections between nerve cells, called *synapses,* where active chemicals are released). Several other nerve centers or *nuclei* also produce dopamine. One, known as the A11 nucleus, sends its axons down the spinal cord where they can make contact with the nerve cells that control the muscles.

The crucial difference between Parkinson's disease (PD) and RLS is that the dopamine shortage in PD results from the death of the cells that produce the neurotransmitter, whereas the dopamine dysfunction that causes RLS is the result of unknown processes and may not even involve an actual overall decrease in dopamine. Moreover, we are not sure if the cells of the SN are responsible for RLS or the cells of one of the other dopamine-making nuclei.

By far the most important dopamine consumer is the *corpus striatum,* in a central area of the brain. The striatum plays a major role in sending out commands for balance and coordination. When you decide to move, whether to hit a golf ball, thread a needle, or extend your middle finger at a careless driver, your commands go from the nigral cells to the striatal cells, from the striatal cells to the spinal cord cells, from the spinal cord cells to the nerve networks, from the nerves to the muscles— all in an instant. The nigral neuron fires dopamine into the striatal neurons by bridging the small gap of the synapse. Dopamine particles speed across the synapse to special pouches called receptors. They have an affinity for a particular neurotransmitter, in this case dopamine. Such receptors are identified, with their subtypes, as D1, D2, D3, D4, and D5. Some of the subtypes are more sensitive to dopaminergic drugs than others, but their precise functions are still imperfectly understood.

Upon the arrival of dopamine, the receiving cell is stimulated to gather its own packets of dopamine and pass the message on to the neighboring nerve cell. Coordination of movement is not only speedy but precise: too much or too little dopamine can disrupt the process, so the receiving cell, having "used" the available dopamine, releases it back into the synapse. This free-floating dopamine, along with any extra that didn't fit in a receptor, is mopped up by a chemical known as MAO-B. In RLS, sensorimotor receptors appear to suffer a shortfall of dopamine; we don't yet know why.

Dopamine doesn't work alone. Several other messengers play an essential role in ensuring smooth muscular movement. The brain regulates or balances the amount of dopamine with another neurotransmitter called acetylcholine. The brain also uses a chemical cousin of dopamine called epinephrine, also known as adrenaline, which is made not only in the brain but in the adrenal gland. Like dopamine, epinephrine also generates emotional responses, including the ability to experience pleasure and pain. Dopamine doesn't have the same ability as adrenaline to create a full-fledged fight-or-flight response, but it's a powerful stimulant when taken in large doses. Dopamine can lower blood pressure when taken in low doses, but paradoxically, in higher doses it is used to keep the blood pressure from dropping in patients who are in shock.

Other substances, like opiates, also affect the receptors involved, but the key element in RLS is dopamine, as it is in PLM. Researchers are divided as to whether a disproportionate number of PD patients get RLS, but they agree that RLS patients do not get PD disproportionately.

Adjusting dopamine processes is no easy matter. "You have to keep in mind," warns Dr. William Ondo, "that whatever you do to change neurotransmitters in the body, the body fights it—always fights it and usually wins. The brain wants to do what it wants to do, and what it wants to do is keep the body in a state of equilibrium."

CURRENT OPTIONS FOR MEDICATION

The following information about medications is offered for patients with RLS and for medical professionals who may want more details about treating the disease. *Patients should not use this information to treat themselves.* They should instead consult a knowledgeable physician. If no informed doctor is within a reasonable distance, you can check with the RLS Foundation's list of doctors treating patients for RLS in Appendix D or on its frequently updated website (www.rls.org). Your doctor may want to use the information below as a guide.

DOPAMINERGIC AGENTS

Dopaminergic agents inhibit abnormal movements by enhancing levels of dopamine. These medications include dopamine precursors and dopamine agonists.

Dopamine precursors are drugs which the body must convert into dopamine first.

Dopamine agonists are drugs that imitate or mimic the action of levodopa in the brain by directly stimulating dopamine receptors, the same receptors that dopamine itself stimulates.

Many RLS patients have a love-hate relationship with the first of the dopaminergic agents, levodopa, which was developed to treat Parkinson's disease. Levodopa, taken in combination with carbidopa (Sinemet), is a dopamine precursor. Carbidopa prevents the levodopa from breaking down in the body before it gets to the brain, where it is needed to treat RLS.

Some people with RLS like dopamine precursors because they usually work and are relatively inexpensive. Physicians may like them because they can be used as a speedy diagnostic tool: if symptoms subside with Sinemet, and if the disease clearly isn't Parkinson's, then the diagnosis of RLS can usually be confirmed. No other dopamine agent provides results so quickly, and it is less expensive than some of the alternatives.

Why is Sinemet also disliked? Because it often has disagreeable side effects (nasal congestion, nausea, sleepiness, and mental confusion are possible) and, more important, because it eventually causes, in about 80 percent of people with RLS, rebound and/or augmentation. (*Rebound* is the intensification and recurrence of symptoms late at night or in the morning as the effects of the drug wear off. *Augmentation* is a two-hour or more time shift of symptoms to an earlier time of day than was typical before the drug was used. Symptoms may also increase in intensity and spread to other parts of the body.) I was in that 80 percent who developed augmentation on Sinemet. At work I would twist in the chair, jiggle my legs, get up and walk—and curse. Day wasn't as bad as night, in part because diversions were available, but it no longer provided a respite.

As more is learned about these medications, doctors are increasingly able to use them selectively to maximize their benefit and limit side effects. A serious possible side effect of dopamine agonists is *sleep attacks*—the sudden onset of sleep, which, if it occurs while the person is operating a motor vehicle or other heavy machinery, may cause an accident. Sleep attacks are not common, however, and almost all have been reported in Parkinsonian patients, who tend to have problems with alertness even without medication. RLS patients also take comparatively small doses of these medications, which may reduce their risk of sleep attacks.

What about Long-Term Effects of Dopaminergics? A cautionary note was heard among researchers as the use of dopaminergic drugs increased. Although those agents are now the treatment of choice for most diagnostician doctors, the concern earlier on, understandably, was over the relatively new drug's long-term effects. I have chosen warnings by two major figures in that field to show how seriously the problem was treated only a few years ago.

Steven E. Hyman, MD, former director of the National Institute of Mental Health, and former member of the RLS Foundation's Scientific Advisory Board, expressed reservations at a workshop in 1999[2]: "The trouble with all the dopaminergic drugs is that there are so many dopamine receptors in the body. It would take a great deal of research and many clinical trials to determine whether any of these other sites of dopamine action may be adversely affected by use of dopaminergic drugs."

A warning was made by Dr. J. Steven Poceta, of the Scripps Clinic and Research Foundation, in an interview with the author:

After determining the target symptom, the next thing in choosing the medication is the age of the patient. I have no favorite drug for

RLS. Doctors who say they always use the same drug, we call that, disparagingly, "cookbook medicine."

I am concerned about the patient's age. If this is a lifelong disorder, and the person is severely affected at age forty, he or she may have this thing for maybe forty more years, I used to hesitate to give that person a dopamine drug, but they are now well-tested and appear to be safe in all age groups.

In contrast to the dopaminergic drugs, the sleeping pills—the benzodiazepines like Valium (diazepam), Klonopin (clonazepam), Restoril (temazepam)—have been around for thirty or forty years. You can take them for a long time and they won't harm you. Yes, you can get addicted to them, they can make you dopey in the morning—there can be side effects, but we're not aware of any really serious long-term complications. And the same is true of codeine.

I have a certain confidence in knowing that the drug has been out there a long time. I'm obviously not as concerned about forty years of exposure for a seventy-year-old patient.

These two cautions have since been modified by the above experts and most others. L-dopa has been used for chronic, lifelong treatments, starting in childhood for dopa-responsive dystonia. L-dopa and the agonists have been used for years for Parkinson's disease. There have been no reports of these problems causing cognitive malfunctions.

BENZODIAZEPINES: SEDATIVES, HYPNOTICS, AND RELATED DRUGS

Some doctors, like Dr. Mark J. Buchfuhrer, make a distinction between "mild intermittent" and "mild persistent" RLS. While preferring nonbenzodiazepines, he sometimes uses the benzodiazepines (central nervous system depressants) when either the nonbenzodiazepines didn't work or were too expensive. He defines "mild" as the occurring of symptoms only at bedtime. Using these RLS medications only intermittently, patients don't need to worry about tolerance or addiction.

For a more persistent form of RLS, Dr. Buchfuhrer prefers a dopamine receptor agonist like Mirapex or Requip. "Side effects of the benzos are quite similar in all the medications in this class. Addiction with tolerance and withdrawal problems can occur with almost all of them, making intermittent use of periodic drug holidays desirable. All the medications should be started at the lowest dose and increased only if necessary."

Among the benzodiazepines, Dr. Buchfuhrer lists Xanax (alprazolam),

> which, although not marketed as a sleeping pill, works quite well in most users to control nighttime RLS problems without much daytime sleepiness. Xanax actually has a half-life of eleven hours, which is likely a little too long but is still much shorter than most of all the other benzos recommended for sleep except Restoril (half-life of about eleven hours) or Halcion. . . . What makes Xanax and Restoril good choices is that they are generic and cheap.

The new sedative/hypnotic Lunesta (eszopiclone), which was just approved, was studied for longer term use than other drugs introduced in the past and was screened for daytime residua. As for Ambien (zolpidem), "It is not a benzodiazepine, but it does work selectively on some of the benzodiazepine receptors." Because of this selectivity, Ambien appears to have fewer side effects than other drugs in this class. It is unique among sedative pills in that does not alter the sleep stages. Most drugs in this class increase stage 2 sleep (a good thing) and decrease sleep stages 1, 3, and 4, and possibly even REM sleep (which might be a bad thing, although this is still not well understood). Ambien also poses no problems with *rebound insomnia*—increased problems falling asleep the night after using the drug. The use of short-acting sedatives like Halcion (triazolam) can cause rebound insomnia or short-term amnesia.

Restoril, which has a longer-than-usual onset of action, is therefore not as good for RLS problems that occur on going to sleep but may be appropriate for RLS and especially PLM that may occur after sleep onset.

Most researchers agree that Klonopin, which was once widely prescribed for RLS and PLM and has a very long half-life (thirty to forty hours), is no longer a drug of choice. Daytime sleepiness and other side effects, including addiction, can be a problem for many patients.

Daytime sleepiness and cognitive impairment, especially in the elderly, are the two most serious possible side effects of the benzodiazepines. All users of benzodiazepines should refrain from the use of alcohol and should not operate motor vehicles or heavy machinery.

NARCOTICS/OPIOIDS AND OTHER ANALGESICS

Because of problems, immediate and potential, with benzodiazepines and dopaminergic agents, some doctors prefer to start their patients with opiates. Others shy away from the opiates because colleagues frown on their use or because of fear that patients will become addicted. It was Dr. Ekbom's view, for example, that the use of narcotics for RLS be restricted to desperate cases. Nonetheless, he wrote that codeine and opium "have a considerably better symptomatic effect than barbiturates," adding that "I have seen certain patients who have taken a narcotic orally every night for years. Some of them did not need to increase the dose."[3]

A study of opioid use for RLS concluded that "opioids can be successfully used long-term with little risk of addiction."[4] In an interview with the author, Dr. Wayne Hening makes the case for the prudent use of opiates in the treatment of RLS and PLM:

There is a definite role for opioids. It depends on the patient, of course, but whole varieties of patients can benefit, as we have seen in a series of studies by Dr. [Arthur] Walters and others—studies showing that opioids can be helpful in RLS and PLM, although less is known about the latter. Those studies involved a mixed population of patients in which opioids were the mainstay of therapy. These patients had been treated for a period of one to fifteen years with only modest increments of dose.

For certain patients the opioids are particularly helpful: First, many people with RLS find there are certain situations where, predictably, they're going to be affected—the theater, dinner party, airplanes—and if it's a reasonably short period, an opiate is a good p.r.n. ("as needed") medication. One can also do that with Sinemet but not, for example, as easily with a dopamine receptor agonist, which may need to be increased slowly to avoid side effects.

Another appropriate use of opioids is with patients who have no sleep problems—people, for example, who only experience leg discomfort in the evening.

Others who can benefit from the use of opioids are those who have a problem with other medications—who can't tolerate benzodiazepines or dopaminergic agents. Opioids can be a good substitute.

Since there many opioids available, from mild to heavy-duty, they may meet the varying needs of patients who are lightly to severely afflicted, as well as the needs of severely afflicted victims who have gone through everything. Opioids can be a good monotherapy for long-term treatment of RLS.

The narcotic analgesics most commonly used for RLS are combined with acetaminophen: Tylenol 3 (with codeine), hydrocodone (Vicodin), and oxycodone (Percocet). Many people on the RLS website have reported being on one of these medications for a number of years.

For patients with intractable disease, when a doctor has established that a variety of other medications, including combination therapies, haven't worked, Dr. Hening and others turn to narcotic analgesics like methadone, levorphanol, extended release oxycodone (OxyContin), morphine (in MS Contin), or fentanyl patches. In rare cases, patients have implanted pumps to deliver narcotics like morphine directly over the spinal cord.

Some narcotic analgesics, like oxycodone, have a shorter half-life, which can cause the rebound or "on and off" phenomenon. Rebound induces some people to take more and more medication, particularly if they have an underlying addictive tendency. However, researchers who have studied the problem say they have rarely seen any of these drugs abused.

One study of opioid use for RLS, conducted by scientists for the journal *Sleep*, concluded that "opioids can be successfully used long term with little risk of addiction."[5] Dr. Bruce L. Ehrenberg, assistant professor of neurology at Tufts University School of Medicine and former chair of the RLS Foundation medical advisory board, found "very little tendency among RLS patients to abuse the opiates or benzodiazepines. More often they are afraid to try them, out of inordinate fear of addiction. People who are prone to addiction have usually declared themselves by the age that most RLS patients first present, and the rate of new-onset addiction in the elderly is quite low."

"People think it is highly risky to give an elderly patient opiates when it is really the opposite," wrote Dr. Charles Cleeland of the

Anderson Cancer Center in a *JAMA* editorial.[6] "Elderly patients can tolerate and need the medicine."

However, as with so many drugs, the hazards of side effects in the elderly (dizziness is more common, for example) may dictate more limited use of opioids and other narcotics. A prudent prescription might call for supplementing lower dosages of drugs from that family with drugs from one or more of the other categories used to combat RLS. Patients should also be carefully screened for sleep apnea, since a small number of patients reporting apneic events developed respiratory irregularities.[7]

Legal issues concerning prescribing narcotics vary by state. "All opiates are carefully controlled," Dr. Walters observes, "but when it comes to methadone, which we use for the most severe cases—cases that don't respond to anything else—physicians are monitored closely."

The use of narcotic analgesics is especially appropriate when arthritis makes nightwalking difficult. Both diseases usually get worse with age, which means that millions of people have a severe form of each. Drugs that are recommended for severe musculoskeletal pain by the Arthritis Foundation include four that can also be of great help to patients with severe RLS who can't take nonsteroidal anti-inflammatory drugs like aspirin or ibuprofen. Those two-way drugs include acetaminophen with codeine (Percocet, Tylenol 3), oxycodone (OxyContin, Roxicodone); hydrocodone with acetaminophen (Vicodin, Lorcet), and tramadol (Ultram).

ANTICONVULSANTS

Two anticonvulsant medications, gabapentin (Neurontin) and carbamazepine (Tegretol), are used to treat RLS. Both drugs have been tested and found to be effective. Although one sleep study concluded that gabapentin was not effective as a treatment for PLM, a later double-blind crossover study reported "a marked reduction in periodic leg movements during sleep."[8] The encouraging report also showed "increased total sleep time, and slow wave sleep, improved sleep efficiency, and decreased stage 1 sleep during gabapentin treatment."

The article's author, Dr. Diego Garcia-Borreguero of Spain, saw gabapentin as a potent agent for treatment of even severe RLS, without the disadvantages of long-term complications of previously favored treatments. But longer investigations will be needed to confirm gabapentin's long-term tolerability.

This class of drugs was designed to deal with epileptic seizures and has not been approved for use during pregnancy.

When Dr. Barbara Phillips, of the University of Kentucky at Lexington, has to abandon Sinemet, she is increasingly likely to use gabapentin, Mirapex, or Requip. "A lot of patients I see with RLS have what I think is a neuropathy. They have diabetes or renal failure, and I just feel that gabapentin works better for those people." Like several other researchers, she finds the anticonvulsant medications especially helpful in cases where pain is involved. Roughly one-third to one-half of patients with mild to moderate RLS appear to respond to the use of gabapentin, with the best response in patients who describe their symptoms as painful. Patients with severe symptoms, however, usually cannot manage with gabapentin alone.

OTHER MEDICATIONS

Ultram (tramadol), a centrally acting synthetic analgesic, is a relatively new painkiller that acts on opiate receptors, although it's not considered part of the opiate family. It is used successfully by itself for RLS or as a medication to substitute when taking a "holiday" from another RLS drug. As is true of many medicines, dosage may have to be reduced for elderly patients to avoid side effects. Like opiates, it can also cause withdrawal problems. The chances of side effects (seizures particularly) are increased if taken with tricyclic antidepressants, selective serotonin reuptake inhibitors, or opioids.

An adrenergic medicine, Catapres (clonidine), developed to treat high blood pressure, has been tested and found to be useful in the treatment of RLS but not PLM. Like Catapres, two other blood pressure medications—Inderal (propranolol) and Cardizem (diltiazem)—have helped a few RLS patients.

POLY, ROTATING, AND COMBINATION THERAPIES

Several physicians, like the pioneering Arthur Walters and Wayne Hening, mix and match treatments. In an interview, Dr. Walters stated he uses drugs from all classes: "For any one patient, there may be a variety of choices that are equally good."

In some cases, Dr. Christopher Earley, of Johns Hopkins, observes, "using a cocktail—two or more drugs at half the previous dose—can produce the benefits seen previously with a larger dose of a single medication, without some of the side effects, and without the early development of tolerance or augmentation." Dr. Earley reviews patients' responses to previous treatment plans to decide which were the most successful. If he decides polytherapy is warranted, he usually selects a dopaminergic agent and an opiate as his first combination. If the patient had a positive response to an anticonvulsant or one of the benzodiazepines, he will use these.

"Trial and error" is an integral part of determining the dosage level as well as whether to use polytherapy, rotating therapy, or combination therapy. In rotating therapy, a single medication is replaced with another every few months. Dr. Earley describes his method:

> I may put patients on a dopamine receptor agonist until they reach either the maximum dose or until they develop tolerance to the medication and have augmentation. Then I substitute another medication, usually a nondopamine agent like an opiate or possibly [a benzodiazepine] clonazepam or [an anticonvulsant] gabapentin. I maintain them on that until they develop tolerance, side effects, or augmentation. I then reinstate the original medication, for example, the dopamine agonist.
>
> Occasionally the rotating therapy will involve a combination therapy. As an example, with a combination of a dopamine agonist and an opiate, one might rotate just the opiate for another opiate or a different class (such as gabapentin).

Such a regimen is challenging for the practitioner, requiring "a sympathetic physician who feels comfortable with the use of the medications."

Again, *never use prescription drugs without the supervision of a physician.* Keep looking until you find a doctor, perhaps a neurologist, who will work as your partner to find the most effective treatment for your RLS.

PHARMACOLOGIC TREATMENT FOR RLS

AGENT	ADVANTAGES	DISADVANTAGES
Dopaminergic agents: dopamine precursor combinations such as carbidopa-levodopa	Can be used on a one-time basis or as circumstances may require. Useful for persons with intermittent RLS because dopamine agonists take longer to have effect.	As many as 80% of patients on carbidopa-levodopa may develop augmentation.* (NOTE: This is at higher doses, >200 mg/day.) Therapeutic effect may be reduced if taken with high-protein food. Can cause insomnia, sleepiness, and gastro-intestinal problems.
Dopamine agonists such as pergolide, pramipexole, ropinirole	Useful in moderate to severe RLS. Recent reports indicate high efficacy of dopamine agonists, but the role of their long-term use is unknown.	Can cause augmentation. Also severe sleepiness, which may limit its use during daytime. Can cause nausea. To avoid this, slow dose increase is important, especially for pergolide.
Opioids such as codeine, hydrocodone, oxycodone, propoxyphene, tramadol	Can be used on an inter-mittent basis. Can also be used successfully for daily therapy.	Can cause constipation, urinary retention, sleepi-ness, or cognitive changes. Tolerance and dependence possible with higher doses of stronger agents.
Benzodiazepines such as clonazepam, temazepam	Helpful in some patients when other medications are not tolerated and may help improve sleep.	Can cause daytime sleepiness and cognitive impairment, particularly in the elderly.

AGENT	ADVANTAGES	DISADVANTAGES
Anticonvulsants such as carbamazepine, gabapentin	Can be considered when dopamine agonists have failed. May be useful in those with coexisting peripheral neuropathy and/or when RLS discomfort is described as pain.	Disadvantages vary depending on agent, but include gastrointestinal disturbance such as nausea, sedation, dizziness.
Iron (ferrous sulfate)	Use in patients with serum ferritin levels <50 mcgL	Ideal means of administration has not been established. Oral treatment may take several months to be effective and may be poorly tolerated.
Clonidine	May be useful in hypertensive patients.	Has the potential to cause hypotension, dermatitis, and sleepiness.

* Augmentation is a worsening of RLS symptoms in the course of therapy. Symptoms may be more severe and start earlier in the day than before treatment began (e.g., afternoon rather than evening) and may spread to different parts of the body. Augmentation, which can start soon after therapy is begun or not until months or years later, has also been reported with dopamine agonists and may occur with other medications.

(From *Restless Legs Syndrome: Detection and Management in Primary Care.* National Center on Sleep Disorders Research and Office of Prevention, Education, and Control. NIH Publication No. 00-3788. March 2000, p. 10.)

AN ALGORITHM FOR DRUG THERAPY

As a result of rapidly increasing knowledge about medications used for RLS, it became possible to create an algorithm—a step-by-step procedure for determining the sequence in which drugs should be tried.[9] The algorithm was devised in 2004 by members of the RLS Foundation's Medical Advisory Board for intermittent, daily, and refractory RLS.

INTERMITTENT RLS troublesome enough when present to require treatment but not frequent enough to necessitate daily therapy.

DAILY RLS frequent and troublesome enough to require daily therapy.

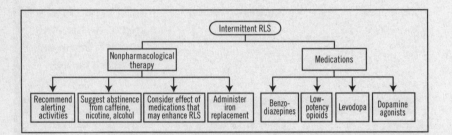

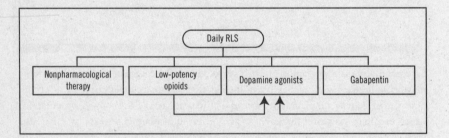

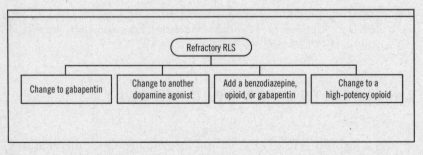

From *Mayo Clinic Proceedings* 2004; 79: 916–22; algorithm produced by Dr. Michael Silber, Dr. Bruce Ehrenberg, Dr. Richard Allen, Dr. Mark Buchfuhrer, Dr. Christopher Earley, Dr. Wayne Hening, and Dr. David Rye.

REFRACTORY RLS daily RLS which when treated with a dopamine agonist produces one or more of the following outcomes:

Inadequate initial response despite adequate doses.

Response that has become inadequate with time, despite increasing doses.

Intolerable adverse effects.

Augmentation that is not controllable with additional earlier doses of the drug.

THE FUTURE OF RLS MEDICATION

As of this writing, the dopamine receptor agonist Requip is the only medication approved by the FDA specifically for treatment of RLS. Like the other agonists, Requip takes between an hour and a half and two hours to work. And as is also true of prescription painkillers, it is less effective if taken after symptoms have started.

A similar medication, pramipexole (Mirapex) is now undergoing clinical trials by Boehringer Ingelheim and may follow ropinirole with approval in 2006 or 2007.

A German company, Schwarz Pharma, which developed a skin patch for treating Parkinson's disease, is conducting clinical trials for the patch's use as a treatment for RLS. Employing a smaller-dose version of the Parkinson's patch provides a sustained delivery of therapeutic levels of medication. Because the drug, rotigotine, already went through intense trials when it was introduced to treat Parkinson's, its use for restless legs moved into second-level government trials more quickly than usual.

Another dopamine agonist, cabergoline, known as Dostinex in the United States, is being investigated in Europe as a possible RLS treatment. It has not been approved by the FDA. A clinical trial of eighty-five patients in Germany concluded that cabergo-line "is an efficacious and well-tolerated option for the treatment of RLS during the night and the day."[10]

Cabergoline has a half-life of sixty-five hours, which could confer an obvious benefit over shorter-acting drugs. In the view of one researcher, however, "it might mask tolerance or augmenta-tion." At its present price cabergoline would cost the average RLS patient about $1,000 a month. Cabergoline's main side effect is se-vere nausea.

Other pharmaceutical companies are actively conducting stud-ies on several different medications for RLS and are certain to fol-low with their own FDA-approved medications.

ANTIDEPRESSANTS AND RLS

Depression is a common problem for victims of RLS, which is scarcely surprising given the sleep deprivation and other stresses ex-perienced by nightwalkers. It is not unusual for doctors to prescribe antidepressants for these cases, but that can be a mistake. Not only do many antidepressants worsen RLS, but some experts believe that certain of the antidepressants are capable of triggering it.

There is strong clinical evidence indicating that virtually all an-tidepressants tend to exacerbate RLS. The old sedating tricyclics—Elavil and Tofranil, for example—appear to be the worst. The newer serotonergic SSRIs, which include Prozac, are also notori-ous for exacerbating nocturnal movements, especially in sleep.

An exception was made by the doctors for Wellbutrin (bupro-pion), also known as Zyban, which is used for smoking cessation. It has an unknown mechanism but, like a few other antidepressants, shows some dopaminergic activity and few side effects. Although

PRESCRIPTION MEDICATIONS USED FOR RLS

BRAND NAME	GENERIC NAME	BRAND NAME	GENERIC NAME
Ambien	zolpidem	Prozac	fluoxetine HCL
Ativan	lorazepam	Reglan	metoclopramide
Cardizem	diltiazem	Requip	ropinirole
Catapres	clonidine	Restoril	temazepam
Depakote	valproate	Roxicodone	oxycodone
Dostinex	cabergoline	Sinemet	carbidopa and levodopa
Elavil	amitriptyline		
Halcion	triazolam	Sonata	zaleplon
Inderal	propranolol	Stadol	butorphanol
Klonopin	clonazepam	Tegretol	carbamazepine
Lioresal	baclofen	Tylenol 3	acetaminophen and codeine
Lorcet	acetaminophen and hydrocodone	Tylox	acetaminophen and oxycodone
Mirapex	pramipexole	Ultram	tramadol
Neurontin	gabapentin	Valium	diazepam
OxyContin	oxycodone	Vicodin	acetaminophen and hydrocodone
Parlodel	bromocriptine		
Percocet	acetaminophen and oxycodone	Wellbutrin	bupropion
Percodan	aspirin and oxycodone	Xanax	alprazolam
Permax	pergolide	Zyban	bupropion

it may not be as useful as some other antidepressants, it is a dopamine agonist and should actually help RLS. (Two of the dopamine agonists, pramipexole and ropinirole, have a slight antidepressant benefit.)

"We prefer to take our RLS patients off antidepressants," said one member of the RLS Foundation Medical Advisory Board, "but these medications are only relatively counterindicated. We certainly have patients on antidepressants whom we are able to treat adequately for their RLS. All classes have been suggested as problems for RLS patients. However, the literature is mixed, because all classes have been reported in some cases to help RLS. My sense is that it is hard to predict in a given case and that you need to try them to find out."

The drug coverage program known as Medicare Part D was launched on January 1, 2006. If you have RLS, or any other chronic condition that requires medication, you should take special care to decide which plan is best for you. Write a list of all the drugs you currently take, even if they are not related to your RLS. Talk to your doctor or specialist about what drugs you might need in the future if your health were to change. Look for a plan that covers the drugs you are currently on and a majority of the drugs it is likely you will need in the future. For more information on RLS and Medicare, visit www.medicare.gov.

ALTERNATIVE MEDICINE

In order to reduce side effects that often occur with the use of levodopa, some doctors combine that dopamine agonist with another drug—usually a neurological agent designed to relax muscles and relieve pain through the nervous system. These alternative therapies permit a reduction in the levodopa dosage while maintaining the benefits of conventional medicines. The physician who prescribes this sort of combined therapy, which may also be identified as holistic, should monitor dosage with more care than is needed for single drug treatment.

Some RLS patients have benefited from acupuncture. One

practitioner, however, dismayed that his daytime treatments of the author seemed to do no good, insisted on trying his skills at night when the RLS was active. As I predicted, the midnight experiment failed because my movements prevented the insertion of needles.

In theory acupuncture stimulates those parts of the brain that are involved in RLS. Some researchers believe that it also reduces the pain of arthritis.

Some RLS patients have reported that they were helped by homeopathy. Homeopaths believe that disorders of the nervous system are especially important because the brain controls so many other bodily functions. Homeopathic remedies are therefore tailored to the individual patient and are based on individual symptoms as well as the general symptoms of RLS.

People who practice reflexology (reflexologists) believe that the brain, head, and spine all respond to indirect massage of specific parts of the feet.

Nutritional supplements are recommended for RLS patients by some doctors. This often involves supplementation of the diet with vitamin E, calcium, magnesium, and folic acid. Herbal therapies, like ginseng, may also be recommended.

Alternative techniques that focus on bodywork, including yoga, may be of special benefit for women for whom pregnancy brought on RLS.

THE ROLE OF IRON

Christopher Earley and his colleague at Johns Hopkins, Richard Allen, PhD, have done comprehensive research on the relationship of RLS and iron. One patient of Dr. Earley's suffered from RLS for nearly six years, with particularly severe symptoms for two or three years preceding her consultation with the Johns Hopkins researcher. "She had gone to many different doctors," he wrote, "and had tried the usual remedies. . . . She had been getting virtually no sleep by the time I saw her and was clearly at her wit's end."

Dr. Earley discovered that his patient's iron and ferritin levels were both abnormally low. This was a significant finding "because ferritin levels are a good indicator of how much iron you have stored and, therefore, how much free iron is available to be utilized by the tissues." (Ferritin is a protein that binds iron. Nature does not want iron running freely around the body, so it provides proteins to which the iron can attach and thus be stored without causing tissue damage.)

After six months of iron supplements, the woman was free of RLS symptoms. To eliminate all symptoms is rare, but Dr. Earley already knew, as do many of his colleagues, that the treatment of iron deficiency may have important clinical benefits for RLS victims.

Since too much iron can be harmful, Dr. Earley cautions his patients to take iron only under a doctor's supervision.

It is telling that a large number—perhaps as many as 25 percent—of RLS patients have iron deficiency. It is also interesting that serum iron levels undergo a daily fluctuation, becoming lowest at night when RLS symptoms are worse.

On hearing about the role of iron in RLS, some victims rush off to ask their doctor for an iron blood test. The doctor may report that the level is OK, not realizing that the serum ferritin level should also be measured. The ferritin test is advisable not only in diagnosing RLS but in monitoring it. The test should be repeated if symptoms worsen. (Ferritin levels below 50 mcg/L may exacer-

IRON AND THE FIRST CLEAR
PHYSICAL MARKER FOR RLS

The first clear clinical evidence of RLS was made possible by the availability of brain tissue obtained from the RLS Foundation Collection at the Harvard Brain Tissue Resource Center. Examination of this tissue showed reduced ferritin and increased transferrin staining in critical motor areas of the brain. Thinking of ferritin units as storage tanks that are used to house iron, and of transferrin as the trucks that deliver iron to nervous system tissue, researchers say that these indicators show that the brain needs iron and is running low on reserves. What isn't clear is why the number of storage tanks is reduced. One possibility is that there is no need to build them since there is not much iron around that needs to be stored. The other possibility is that the iron is there but this area of the brain fails to provide the storage tanks. It may be that both explanations are correct.

Although scientists are pleased with the discovery of the first clear physical marker for RLS, they are confronted with some difficult questions. For example, how does iron penetrate the blood-brain barrier in some people—those who don't have RLS—and why does less pass through for RLS victims? Is it possible to circumvent the brain barrier with iron given through the veins? Even more difficult: What chemical role does iron play in the complicated dopamine system?

bate RLS symptoms even though such levels are still within the normal range, which may go down to 10 or 18 mcg/L.)

The relationship between RLS and iron deficiency was first noted by Nordlander (1953) and later verified by Ekbom (1960).[11] Further research indicates that altered iron metabolism within the central nervous system (CNS) may play a significant role in RLS.

One study by Allen and Earley found that in RLS patients, CNS ferritin levels were abnormally low in the cerebrospinal fluid that bathes the brain and spinal cord—even when serum ferritin and iron levels were normal. Thus, transport of iron across the blood-brain barrier, or the way the CNS handles iron, may be one of the deficiencies in this disorder. In an interview with the author, Dr. Richard Allen explains what makes this finding so relevant "is that iron is a cofactor with tyrosine hydroxylase, the rate-limiting step in the production of dopamine, and it is dopamine agonists that are the cornerstone of therapy in RLS." In other words, iron is essential for the production of dopamine, and if iron is low, dopamine may not function normally.

RLS IN END-STAGE RENAL DISEASE (ESRD)

Two secondary "causes" of RLS, kidney failure (ESRD) and pregnancy, are associated with iron deficiency. And it has been noted clinically that rates of RLS in dialysis patients appear to have decreased with aggressive use of iron given by the vein. But more research is needed, as evidenced by the failure in two studies to find a relationship between iron indices and RLS in patients with kidney failure.[12]

Such research goes beyond academic interest: more than half of those undergoing the blood-cleaning procedure known as dialysis—which extends lives but drains patients of money, time, and energy—will experience the urge to move their limbs. But because they are tethered to tubes and pumps and filtering devices, they cannot avail themselves of the best remedy—walking.

That this is a serious issue is evident in the following numbers: more than 50,000 Americans die each year because of kidney disease, more than 260,000 Americans suffer from chronic kidney failure and require dialysis or kidney transplantation, and more than 48,000 patients are waiting for kidney transplants.[13] The cause of the prevalence of RLS and PLM among dialysis patients is not yet understood, but current estimates are that 25 to 40 percent of dialysis patients suffer from RLS. The disease does not appear to be caused by the procedure itself, because it frequently develops before the patient needs dialysis. The villain appears to be kidney failure. For example, RLS can be eliminated by kidney transplantation.

RLS and PLM have been associated with both poor treatment compliance and an increased death rate in patients with ESRD. The statistics are startling, writes Dr. John Winkelman:

We documented a nearly twofold relative risk of a history of premature sign-offs [people who give up treatment] in such patients compared to those without RLS.

It is unclear whether the poor treatment compliance accounts for, or is merely associated with, the findings of an elevated death rate in ESRD patients who have either RLS or PLM. In our study of 204 ESRD patients, we demonstrated that those with RLS had a 20 percent higher mortality risk three years after initial evaluation than those without RLS.

Another preliminary report found that the severity of PLM (RLS was not investigated) was a better predictor of mortality in ESRD than comorbid medical disease.

Treatment of the RLS/ESRD patient is generally the same as in those with normal renal function. Correction of underlying causes is the first goal, so in most cases dopaminergic drugs should be tried, with opiates, benzodiazepines, and anticonvulsants being employed as alternatives. Small doses of oxycodone or codeine can be of value for middle-of-the-night or predialysis dosing. Benzodiazepines can be of value in cases where the dopaminergic medications alleviate the restlessness but do not optimize sleep quality. Finally, anticonvulsants are also effective in some dialysis patients, particularly those with painful RLS. Caution should be exercised when using gabapentin, however, as it is cleared solely by the kidneys.[14]

In sum, the nephrologist should not accept poor sleep as inevitable in patients with ESRD. RLS and PLM are a common affliction among them, diagnosis is generally not difficult, and treatment is relatively straightforward.

RLS AND PREGNANCY

It was Ekbom who discovered that a significant number of pregnant women experience RLS and PLM, most during the third trimester. The Swedish neurologist set the prevalence rate at 11.3 percent, noting that in some cases the affliction was new; in other cases existing RLS and PLM worsened.[15] Recent studies show RLS/pregnancy prevalence rates ranging from 11 to 33 percent, with PLM rates at 37 to 40 percent.

Iron and folate deficiency have been mentioned as possible causes, along with anemia, hormonal changes, and vascular congestion. One expert, Dr. Christopher Earley, believes the issue is nutrient deficiency: "The fetus takes all the iron and folic acid and so forth. You can often avoid RLS in pregnancy with high-dose folic acid and iron and vitamin supplements. We absolutely saw iron deficiency and a correlation with symptoms when we replenished patients' iron stores. Their symptoms got dramatically better—both their RLS and the PLM."

Many women suffer the symptoms of RLS and PLM during pregnancy, but few mention them to their doctor or obstetric caregiver, perhaps partly because they have more riveting concerns about their health or the health of their fetus; they may also feel embarrassed about mentioning their inability to sit still. Also, as with many nightwalkers, they may feel, often correctly, that their doctor won't know what they're talking about. If you are pregnant, consult a physician before taking vitamin supplements or medications for RLS.

The most complete epidemiologic study of RLS as it occurs during pregnancy was made public in 2004 by researchers at the Sleep Disorders Center at Vita-Salute University Milan. The study, which included up to six months postpartum, showed that nearly 25 percent of participants developed RLS symptoms during pregnancy.

About 10 percent of those women, as Dr. Bruce Ehrenberg points out in the August 1997 issue of *NightWalkers,* will experience RLS symptoms for the first time in their lives.[16] It would not be unusual for such women to feel "creepy-crawly" sensations or RLS in their legs in the evening or night at the same time they are plagued by fatigue, headaches, and other classic accompaniments of pregnancy.

In any event, it would be wise for a patient to describe all such symptoms to her doctor. She may be dismayed to discover, if she had RLS before pregnancy, that the symptoms are quite severe. The likely explanation is that one or more of the woman's regular medications were halted to protect the fetus. The change may also be caused by hormonal changes or other stress factors.

The use of vitamin and mineral supplements by pregnant women with RLS is approved by most obstetric caregivers. The most important of these supplements are iron, magnesium, vitamin B_{12}, and folate. Of these the most important is folate, the use of which reduces the possibility of birth defects.

Some experts recommend taking iron and magnesium together to reduce possible side effects: constipation in the case of iron, diarrhea in the case of magnesium.

If the use of dopaminergic agents is vetoed because of possible adverse effects on the fetus, one alternative is low-potency opiates. Their advantage, taken in acceptable amounts, is that they don't have a deleterious effect on the fetus. The downside is the possibility of a withdrawal problem in the postpartum period.

Recent advances in the safe use of sleep medicines during pregnancy have largely reduced the discomforts of that condition when aggravated by RLS and PLM. (Also in 2004 the RLS Foundation published the booklet "Pregnancy and RLS: Vital considerations in treating a patient who has restless legs syndrome.")

Very little research to date has been directed at the treatment of RLS in pregnancy. The medications that have proved useful in treating RLS in the general population are nearly all contraindicated in pregnancy. Using the FDA classification system of categories A, B, C, D, and X—with A representing lowest risk and X representing highest risk of teratogenicity—the information below outlines treatments commonly used for RLS and their risk in pregnancy.

DOPAMINERGICS

levodopa/carbidopa (Sinemet, others): *class C.* There is very limited data in human pregnancy, but both levodopa and combinations of carbidopa and levodopa have caused visceral and skeletal malformations in laboratory animals (rabbits).
pramipexole (Mirapex): *class C.* Limited data. Dopaminergic medications inhibit prolactin release, which diminishes lactation.

BENZODIAZEPINES

clonazepam (Klonopin): *class D.* Benzodiazepines can cause neonatal withdrawal syndrome when taken late in pregnancy. The benzodiazepine family of drugs is considered to increase the potential risk of birth defects, fetal dependency, and floppy baby syndrome (an abnormal condition of newborns and infants manifest by inadequate tone of the muscles) after birth or while nursing.

temazepam (Restoril): *class X*. Temazepam with diphenhydramine (Benadryl) has been reported to result in an increased rate of stillbirths.

OPIOIDS

codeine (various products, including Tylenol 3): *class C; class D* if use is chronic.

hydrocodone (Vicodin): *class C; class D* if use is chronic.

propoxyphene (Darvon): *class C; class D* if use is chronic.

oxycodone (OxyContin): *class B; class D* if use is chronic.

Drugs of the opioid class can cause neonatal withdrawal syndrome when taken late in pregnancy. Opioids are excreted in breast milk and thereby can cause sedation in the breast-fed infant.

methadone (Dolophine, Methadose): *class B/C; class D* if dosage is high. While no increase in congenital defects has been observed, low birth weight, neonatal withdrawal, and possible elevated risk for sudden infant death syndrome (SIDS) have been concerns. There is considerable data on methadone use during pregnancy. The transfer of methadone into human milk is minimal, and methadone is considered compatible with breast-feeding.

OTHERS

clonidine (Catapres): *class C*. Inadequate studies in humans. Is excreted in breast milk.

gabapentin (Neurontin): *class C*. Fetotoxic in rodents; inadequate data in humans.

zolpidem (Ambien): *class B*. This medication is excreted in breast milk and should not be taken while nursing.

VITAMINS AND MINERALS

folate: *class A*. An essential nutrient often used during pregnancy as part of a multivitamin preparation.

Iron: *class A*. An essential nutrient often used during pregnancy as part of a multivitamin preparation.

magnesium: *class B*. An essential nutrient used during pregnancy to treat eclampsia and premature labor. Some evidence indicates that magnesium may help RLS.

To receive up-to-date, evidence-based information on the safety and risk of drugs during pregnancy, consult an information service such as Motherisk (motherisk.org), perinatology.com, or the Organization of Teratology Information Services (http://orpheus .ucsd.edu/ctis/).

Alternative Treatment There are few conventional therapies available to pregnant women, since most of the drugs prescribed are not recommended for use during pregnancy. These patients may benefit from alternative techniques that focus on bodywork, including yoga, reflexology, and acupuncture.

CHAPTER 6

More Sources of Help

All for one; one for all.

—Alexandre Dumas, père, *The Three Musketeers*

SUPPORT GROUPS

Support groups provide the two elements most needed by despairing RLS sufferers, hope and help. For Thelma Bradt of Bradenton, Florida, the first coordinator of the RLS Foundation's support group network, having a support group was "the most richly rewarding experience of my life. I don't believe I've ever left a meeting when I haven't mentioned to my husband that I felt so good. It seems we always have one new member visiting us who knows absolutely nothing about the help that is available."

For the most severely afflicted, and for those who suffered, without sympathy or relief, perhaps for decades, such groups can serve as lifeboats. At the very least, they are a source of comfort and information. People get the opportunity to share their stories, compare symptoms, discuss which medicines work, and talk about the coping mechanisms they have tried. Support group members find great relief in knowing they are no longer alone.

A few groups were formed even before the creation of the RLS Foundation in 1992. The need was great, so soon there were dozens of groups, and at the time of this writing there are nearly a hundred in the United States alone. Internationally, active groups can be found in Australia, Austria, Canada, England, Finland, Germany, Holland, New Zealand, and Switzerland.

The most important role of the support group is to demonstrate that RLS is a real and treatable disorder, that others have the same problem, and that neither you nor they are crazy. RLS patients become convinced that they alone have those odd and unsettling symptoms. Many have believed, sometimes because of misguided doctors' diagnoses, that they were deranged.

Loneliness can be a brutal accomplice of RLS. Joining a support group can help banish it. All support groups provide understanding and companionship that is too often unavailable elsewhere, even from friends and relatives.

When people find out what ails them, they want to know whether medications or alternative therapies will help. A support group provides an excellent way of finding out what treatments others have tried. The morale of nightwalkers is palpably improved at meetings where the latest medical strategies are discussed. Group members pick up anecdotal information about RLS: while one member may find some relief through a new drug combination, another may be helped by taking vitamin E and magnesium. While one may get more sleep by taking a hot bath at bedtime, another may tame symptoms by doing deep knee bends.

Many support group participants join the RLS Foundation, thereby becoming subscribers to the excellent *NightWalkers* newsletter, in which they learn about research programs, scientific papers, and new treatments. No less important, membership in the foundation provides a sense of belonging to a growing international venture. The organization acts as a clearinghouse of information for local groups and encourages members to keep their physicians updated on new treatment options.

One benefit of membership in any support group is the knowledge that you will be helping others. The thought that other nightwalkers may find relief as a result of your efforts is not only psychologically rewarding but also a good way of converting self-pity into constructive benevolence.

Most RLS support groups have a medical adviser who is called upon when questions arise about RLS symptoms or treatments. A medical professional may also be able to provide a bonus—a meeting site within his or her health care facility. Mark Buchfuhrer, MD, has been the medical adviser for the Southern California Support Group since its formation in 1996. Going beyond the role of the typical medical adviser, Dr. Buchfuhrer maintains the support group's website (www.rlshelp.org), which contains several pages of frequently asked questions.

"It's really helpful for physicians treating RLS to go to meetings," says Dr. Buchfuhrer, adding that he has gained insights that he wouldn't have from his private practice. "It's a great opportunity for a physician who wants to be more of an expert. Invaluable experience is gained by listening to, and talking with, hundreds of people around the world who are afflicted with RLS/PLM."

The Southern California RLS Support Group illustrates what one such organization can accomplish. It was started by Elizabeth Tunison, a Whittier College professor who has suffered from RLS since childhood. She recalls her mother sitting with her in the back row of church on Sunday nights "so that I could get up and walk around during the sermon. My dad, who was the preacher and also had RLS, didn't have as much of a problem because he didn't have to sit still." It was decades before Professor Tunison discovered, in the course of a major back operation, that drugs given for her post-operative pain also relieved restless legs.

Professor Tunison heard about a sleep clinic run by Dr. Buchfuhrer, to whom she took all her tests and reports from other doctors. "He listened, he understood, and he helped. Together we found medications and a lifestyle that worked best for me."

With the encouragement of Pickett Guthrie, founding executive director of the fledgling RLS Foundation, and the help of Dr. Buchfuhrer and friends, Professor Tunison started the group. She later recalled the first meeting, at which "we were amazed to find so many others who had those same indescribable sensations. We had not known others who understood our misery until that meeting." The first encounter "was tearful, as members told of sleepless nights and of being told by doctors and friends that they were crazy."

That support group flourished, raising funds and awareness with an ocean cruise, greeting-card and videotape sales, a comprehensive website, and a 122-page booklet about RLS and PLM medications and alternative treatments.

Readers who would like to join a support group can contact the RLS Foundation or visit its website at www.rls.org to see whether a group meets in their community. (See also Appendix B.) Readers who can't find a local group may want to join the RLS Cyberspace Support group (www.mlists.net/judson/RLSINTRO). It is run by Jodi Judson, an RLS sufferer for most of her life. This group exchanges messages every day about personal experiences with RLS and treatments.

The foundation sponsors regional and national meetings, sends representatives to national and international medical conferences, and stays in touch with support groups in other countries. In this way, members can feel part of, and contribute to, a worldwide movement that provides solace, help, and hope to millions of RLS patients.

THE ADMIRABLE RLS FOUNDATION

In 1989 a ninety-one-year-old journalist, Oron F. Hawley, began correspondence with eight other long-suffering people with RLS. In the course of letter and telephone exchanges they discovered that they weren't imagining nocturnal troubles, they weren't crazy, they were not alone, and that a few—but just a few—medical researchers were learning about the disease.

Hawley was joined by Pickett Guthrie and Virginia Wilson to form, in November 1992, the Restless Legs Syndrome Foundation. The two women, themselves RLS patients, alternated as president and executive director.

The foundation received tax-exempt status in January 1993. Pickett and Virginia enlisted not only a board of directors but a Medical Advisory Board (MAB) in 1993. They chose medical volunteers of such expertise and stature that the present MAB, built on their enterprise, is widely admired for its contributions to sensorimotor and sleep research.

In May 1994 the IRLSSG (International Restless Legs Syndrome Study Group) and the foundation organized the first international symposium on RLS in Florence, Italy. A Scientific Advisory Board (SAB) was named in 1997. Its first chair was Bruce Alberts, president of the National Academy of Sciences. By the beginning of this century, the foundation maintained a network of nearly a hundred support groups.

The RLS Foundation participates in discussions of RLS at medical conferences. It provides a toll-free number (1-877-463-6757), which anyone can call to receive a complimentary copy of the booklet *Living with Restless Legs*.

It maintains a busy and comprehensive website at www.rls

.org, responding to e-mail messages from RLS patients, from their puzzled friends and relatives, and from doctors and nurses. The site also contains a frequently-asked-questions (FAQ) section and an intriguing collection of letters.

The RLS Foundation funds research through a competitive grants program devoted to identifying the cause of RLS, developing effective treatments for the disease, and finding a cure. It seeks to increase the number of scientists who are studying RLS by funding fellowship awards. It also maintains the RLS Foundation Collection at the Harvard Brain Tissue Resource Center, to provide postmortem tissue for research scientists.

The RLS Foundation has played an important role in many lives, including that of Margarette Fuhr of Boulder, Colorado, who became a board member. Marge has had RLS since she was a teenager. Over the years, she tried many medications in her search for relief.

> The first real breakthrough came when my youngest son discovered the RLS Foundation on the Internet. I immediately wrote to them and was sent information. I vividly remember reading the little pamphlet they sent, which described RLS symptoms in such a way that I thought they were describing me. The relief, the sense that someone else understands, the knowledge that RLS isn't "in my head," the realization that I was not alone brought tears to my eyes.
>
> Now I'm a board member of the organization that profoundly changed my life. It brought me solace and hope. I trust that my work will bring the same sort of solace and hope to uncounted victims of a vicious disease.

The speedy growth of the RLS Foundation necessitated hiring a professional staff, but volunteers still perform many of the essential tasks. Volunteers include a board of directors, all of whom suffer from RLS or have family members who do.

Meetings of the board, consequently, involve a great deal of restless movement. A stranger walking into the conference room would be startled at the sight of board members jiggling their legs, pacing the room, and occasionally doing deep knee bends. During intermissions, the stranger would overhear conversations largely concerned with how well the members and others had slept the night before.

The work of the RLS Foundation changes lives, for example that of Laura Schmidt from Garland, Texas. She consulted Dr. Philip M. Becker, a former member of the Medical Advisory Board of the RLS Foundation and medical director of the Sleep Medicine Institute in Dallas, Texas.

When I went to see Dr. Becker, I brought a page-long list of medications that I had tried for RLS. He systematically went through my rather long history and discussed it with my husband and me. . . . It was great to be an active partner in my care. He listened carefully while we described how RLS and PLM had brought me to the point where I was not able to work anymore. I had restricted my activities to the point where I *had no life!*

As a result of Dr. Becker's advice, I recovered a majority of my life (with some restrictions). He suggested a medication that he uses only for those cases where nothing else has worked. My symptoms are now minimal. I consistently sleep six to eight hours a night. I can go to the movies or the theater and have even flown across country.

I have not been able to return to work yet but am hoping to try part-time.

Dr. Richard Levin asserts that "the best way to make doctors more aware of RLS is to have informed patients ask specific questions. This is where the RLS Foundation plays an important role, along with the various sleep associations and the lay media. As victims become familiar with their illness through such organizations, they will spur doctors to investigate. They will also make use of information available on the Internet."

Thousands of RLS patients have found out what they have, and what to do about it, by looking up the disease on the Internet. At the RLS Foundation's website, you can, for a small sum, become a member and thereby obtain the following benefits:

- *NightWalkers,* the Foundation's quarterly newsletter, in which physicians, scientists, and patients write about the latest treatments and research findings. *NightWalkers* summarizes articles published in medical journals, reports on research results presented at medical meetings, and answers questions that readers put to members of the Medical Advisory Board. The newsletter also carries articles about foundation and support group activities. No less important and interesting are letters from readers about their trials and triumphs in living with RLS.
- A *Medical Bulletin and Bibliography* to educate health care professionals.
- An information booklet, *Living with Restless Legs.*
- A medical alert card listing symptoms of RLS.
- Enrollment of your health care provider in the foundation's database, which provides an annual mailing of the *Medical Bulletin and Bibliography* to the health care provider.
- Access to the foundation's physician referral program, which provides members with the names of doctors who are aware of RLS treatments.
- Information about newly formed RLS support groups.
- Free shipping and handling of foundation materials.

• A pamphlet, *Restless Legs Syndrome: A Guide for the Perioperative Team*, for anesthesiologists, surgeons, and nurses.

This last item addresses the problem for nightwalkers of enforced inactivity after surgical procedures. The agony of such inactivity is likely to be remembered longer and more vividly than the surgical procedures themselves.

The pamphlet describes RLS, identifies its primary features, and lists substances that may be useful in treating the disease. (It also identifies substances that should *not* be given to RLS patients, including neuroleptic agents, dopamine blockers, and certain antidepressants and antiemetic agents.)

Patients scheduled for an operation, who are taken off their usual medications, should give a copy of the pamphlet to their surgeon well in advance of the event. Many surgical team members are unfamiliar with RLS and therefore unaware of the discomfort it can inflict on its victims. This is particularly true, as the pamphlet points out, "in the immediate postoperative period when quiescence often exacerbates the need to move."

The pamphlet does not say, but I shall, that failure to use RLS therapy in hospitals has resulted in patients' intense agitation. Some plagued patients have had to be restrained after trying to crawl over hospital bed railings. Postoperative immobilization, pain, and sleep deprivation can worsen symptoms and lengthen recovery. A failure to heed such advice may interfere with the operation itself, particularly when periodic leg movements occur.

It is impressive that in only one decade the RLS Foundation has changed the lives of countless RLS sufferers. Few, if any, citizen-based nonprofit organizations devoted to a medical problem have expanded as rapidly as the RLS Foundation. It merits the praise and help it has received from the National Institutes of

Health, the National Academy of Sciences, and other scientific bodies.

The letter writers had no way of knowing how much help they were providing themselves by calling attention to the large number of RLS patients, to the seriousness of the disease, and to the need for a book of this sort. Those letters became the taproot of the RLS Foundation, which "is dedicated to improving the lives of men, women, and children who live with this often devastating disease. The organization's goals are to increase awareness of restless legs syndrome, to improve treatments, and through research, find a cure." They unwittingly provided a mutual assistance that was eventually to be found in support groups.

Oron Hawley, pioneer, would surely be impressed and optimistic about the foundation's future. In 2005 Robert H. Waterman Jr., coauthor of *In Search of Excellence*, ended a busy six-year term as chairman of the RLSF board. In that time the Scientific Advisory Board was formed, links forged with the National Institutes of Health, research projects tripled, and membership doubled.

An equally energetic board member, Lew Phelps, was elected to replace Waterman in 2006. Phelps successfully streamlined foundation activities by employing technology used in his public relations firm. One product of this technological advance was the RLS Website Community, located at www.rls.org. Designed to improve communications with the public, it also provides services for members, including access to publications, a searchable database, and even photo albums of events.

PARTNERSHIP WITH THE NIH

People who created the RLS Foundation in 1992 knew that it could more quickly reach its goals (achieving universal awareness, identifying better treatment, finding a cure) by working with the National Institutes of Health (NIH). They also knew that such an association would help the NIH reach *its* goals—to help prevent, detect, diagnose, and treat disease and disability. But there was a big problem: the NIH didn't know the RLS Foundation existed. Some NIH staff members didn't even know there was such a disease.

The RLS Foundation realized that legions of sufferers could be helped if the world's foremost medical research center joined in the effort to understand and treat RLS. How should the nascent foundation go about making an alliance with the government's primary health agency?

The task of selling the NIH on the need for a mutual assistance program fortunately fell largely to Robert Balkam, a nightwalker and foundation board member. Balkam was aided by foundation officials, especially Robert Waterman, then chairman of the RLS Foundation's board of directors, and Carolyn Hiller, then the foundation's executive director. Balkam's job was also strengthened by the RLS Foundation's impressive medical and scientific advisory boards, made up of doctors whose names were likely to be familiar to NIH officials.

Given NIH ignorance of RLS, Balkam's task was daunting: to familiarize the NIH with the prevalence of the disease and to demonstrate the urgent need for research on the causes of RLS.

In February 1997 Balkam and foundation colleagues worked with Bruce Alberts, president of the National Academy of Sciences. Alberts arranged a meeting at his organization's headquarters, where for the first time clinicians who were treating RLS met with basic scientists, many of whom had never heard of the disease.

On the delicate subject of research funding, Balkam informed NIH staff that the foundation was prepared to do its part. In Balkam's view, "Too many grant-seeking groups expect the NIH to do it all." The foundation proposed, and the NIH accepted, a research project on RLS prevalence largely funded and organized by the RLSF newcomers. The research funds came from a thin budget, but the expenditure was worth it.

The NIH now understood that many Americans would suffer in the absence of research leading to better treatment of RLS and PLM. One measure of the change in relations between the RLS Foundation and the NIH is seen in an increasing number of intra-mural grants for RLS/PLM research. A search of the NIH data-base for the years 1990–97 reveals a mere three grants that included the term *restless legs syndrome*. A December 18, 2005, search of the NIH database for RLS studies showed 12 grants.

As a measure of the NIH's increasing interest in RLS, in 1999, NIH's Dr. Charlotte McCutchen organized a workshop called The Dopamine Connection that brought together major scientific figures, including Bruce Alberts; Dr. Steven Hyman, then director of the National Institute of Mental Health, currently chancellor of Harvard; Dr. Michael J. Brownstein of National Institute of Mental Health, also a member of the RLSF's Scientific Advisory Board; Dr. Gerald Fischbach, then director of National Institute of Neurological Disorders and Stroke and presently vice president for health and biomedical sciences at Columbia University; Dr. Mark Hallett of NINDS and vice president of the American Academy of Neurology; and many other distinguished scientists. Currently the NIH sponsors or cosponsors twenty-five RLS studies.

The NIH has shown what a government agency can do, work-ing with volunteer patient organizations like the RLS Foundation, to improve citizens' health. Millions of RLS victims will benefit. No precise statistics will be available, of course, but we can be con-fident that ten years from now there will be fewer suicides, fewer accidents, fewer jobs lost, fewer tormented nights, fewer dysfunc-tional families, thanks to these efforts.

CHAPTER 7

Coping

But if you try sometimes . . .
You get what you need.

—MICK JAGGER AND KEITH RICHARDS

Over the years, like other panicky nightwalkers, I would experiment to find relief. At one time or another, I tried hot water
(nearly scalding), icy water (nearly freezing), sleeping pills
(which made walking harder), and acupuncture. The acupuncturist
was so intrigued by the challenge that he offered to continue my
sessions free. He even came to my house at midnight in an effort,
altogether unsuccessful, to stop the RLS at its worst. The acupuncturist couldn't even place the needles, so great was my need to move
at that time of night.

Stretching relieved the symptoms, as did deep knee bends, but
not for long. Slapping or punching my legs provided a temporary if
masochistic respite. Occasionally I expunged the sensation by lying
on my back and "cycling," but no one could keep that up for long.
Nor could my wife, Alice, tolerate such activity for more than a few
minutes. I am only slightly ashamed to admit that now and then I
cried. I believe that most sufferers of severe RLS do.

Alice, who thinks she has insomnia if she isn't asleep in five minutes, would be breathing regularly, a book lying on her chest, and an expression of contentment on her face. She always looks as though she enjoys sleep, actually smiling some of the time. I tried not to notice as I *walked* by.

REMEDIES FROM A TO Z

Nearly every vitamin, mineral, medication, prayer, diet, holistic practice, and exercise routine has been tried by nightwalkers, or by their doctors, in efforts to alleviate RLS symptoms. Indeed, attempts at remedies for RLS and PLM range from aspirin and acupuncture to zinc and zodiac consultations. In desperation, sufferers have tried almost everything. Some methods work temporarily by means of the placebo effect; some actually make a certain amount of scientific sense.

One woman wrote that putting a fabric softener in the foot of her stockings helped. Another wrote about "a biomagnetic product" consisting of "a very thin insole with magnets which react with the positive and negative ions in the blood." Yet another sufferer informed the Southern California Support Group that she had trumped the scientific community by identifying the cause of RLS: "I'm a trained psychic and healer and when I look at the energy of this syndrome, I see one thing, one cause, regardless of what name is used for it or whether it's arms or legs, daytime or nighttime. The cause is lack of grounding. The body is not connected adequately to the planet, so that your energy flow is blocked, and blocked energy causes restlessness, jumpiness, irritation, twitchiness, tingliness, and eventually pain and physical disease or illness."

Heat and cold are favorite themes. Many people run hot or cold water over their legs for temporary relief. Ernest Barth, a night-walker from Pierre, South Dakota, actually welcomes winter because he can stand in the snow: "I know all about walking at night. I have been out as late as 2 a.m. in the winter (and in South Dakota that is misery magnified to the nth degree)." Mary E. Higgins of Kingston, Tennessee, prefers very hot baths.

At least one nightwalker found success with bandages: "I have found one thing that helps [my RLS]. I have two Ace bandages. I start about middle of the leg between knee and hip and wrap my legs like a flagpole—as tight as I can wrap them without cutting off the circulation. I wrap them below the knees. Believe me, this has given me lots of nights' sleep that I would not have had. If I start getting the restless legs again, I unwrap them and they will ease off."

Another tried wrapping her legs in Ace bandages "every night for a year." That apparently didn't work for her, however, so she reported trying aspirin, quinine, Tylenol, ibuprofen, diazepam, baclofen, Permax, Sinemet regular and CR, Klonopin, calcium carbonate and citrate, magnesium, potassium, and vitamin E.

"I tried taking megadoses of vitamins," another nightwalker reports. "I tried no vitamins. I tried vigorous exercise—no exercise. I tried hot baths—no hot baths. I tried (endured) ice and cold baths—no ice and cold baths. I even tried using a sewing needle to poke my legs, thinking, in my little pea brain, that I could somehow 'distract' the RLS. Of course, none of that worked. The only answer was to walk and walk and walk."

Sometimes relief comes in strange guises. A woman from El Monte, California, reported, "I had RLS very bad for years but not anymore." She had broken her hips. "My doctor ordered a trapeze for me so I could get in and out of bed easier . . . I would lie on my

back with both feet in the swing and swing for at least thirty minutes several times a day." Her restless legs went away. Another offered this advice: "Take iron tablets or make yourself a drink with
blackstrap molasses and one tablespoon of honey, hot water, and
half-and-half. . . . I'm eighty-seven years old and am doing fine."

Dianne Phillips of Memphis, Tennessee, tried wearing a cast
on one leg "to see if immobilization would help." It didn't. "The
physical therapist tried some sort of boot with intermittent pressure to see if circulation was the problem." It wasn't. She "finally
gave up on doctors and tried to learn to live with my symptoms."
Others have tried propping their legs up against a wall or kneeling
in prayer position by the bed until their feet and legs are numb.

All sorts of suggestions for relief appear in the lively RLS chat
rooms. One participant reported having surgery for varicose veins.
"I naively thought my RLS symptoms might be alleviated by the
surgery. Everyone should be very careful before you let any doctor
fool with your legs." Describing how the RLS returned far worse
than before, she said: "If I had the choice to make again, I would
not have had the surgery."

It was once not unreasonable for some patients and researchers
to think that the source, or one of the sources, of RLS lay in the
traitorous legs themselves. Ekbom and some others believed that
RLS was linked to vascular disease. One doctor announced in *Dermatologic Surgery* (1995) that compression sclerotherapy, which involves injecting a solution into a vein to shrink it, resulted in 98
percent of patients becoming asymptomatic after three or fewer
treatments.[1] Although this much optimism over a surgical procedure turned out to be unwarranted, there are some researchers who
cite enough anecdotal evidence to justify studies of circulatory
problems and RLS. Vascular disorders have been listed in scientific
articles as an associated feature of RLS.

In the search for a do-it-yourself remedy, few nightwalkers have been as inventive as John Williams of Baton Rouge, Louisiana:

I am a beekeeper. The venom you receive when you are stung is a protein. If you get too many stings, you faint because the protein causes the lining of the blood vessels to relax so they don't help pump the blood back. Since movement helped relieve RLS, I thought the solution might be circulatory. Maybe RLS needs help in getting the blood back out and moving.

So one night when I had it especially bad, I went to the backyard, put my hand up in the beehive, and got stung several times in order to get that venom in my bloodstream. But it didn't do any good.

I tried another thing about 3:30 one morning. I had shaken and tensed and stretched and jumped up and down with the RLS. I had been working on engines a bit and I had been shocked by an internal combustion engine. Being desperate, I went out, attached a wire to one of my spark plug wires, and laid it on the ground. Holding on to the insulated part, I took a very light wire and wrapped it around my legs. Then, putting one foot on the bumper and the other on the ground, I touched the spark plug wire. I was shocked, but the RLS was unaffected.

You become so frustrated in the middle of the night that you say, I don't care if it kills me or not.

Williams later heard that RLS could be assuaged by tarantula urine or by marijuana dissolved in alcohol used as lotion. But he couldn't report on them because by then he had decided to shun unconventional treatments.

THE SEARCH FOR DIVERSIONS

Many nightwalkers find relief in distracting themselves with mental and physical activity. "Relax" can be the worst advice. Margarette Fuhr tried a variety of relaxation techniques, including yoga and massage:

> I learned that moments of relaxation are exactly the times that RLS loves to attack its victims. RLS stalks me even at the end of a yoga class. The symptoms come on when I sit down to read a book or watch TV or settle in for the night. I couldn't even enjoy a full body massage because I couldn't keep still.
>
> This peculiarity—the evoking of symptoms while at rest—is the hardest for others to understand. Well-meaning friends encourage you to be calm, to relax, and to have positive thoughts. But sometimes the opposite of being relaxed can bring relief. Emotional involvement or absorption in an activity, like playing the piano or writing at the computer, can sometimes alleviate symptoms. A woman at a support group said she could often find relief while playing poker.

Some nightwalkers strap on a portable cassette player and listen to books on tape. Others watch television while walking on a treadmill. It isn't easy, but some treadmillers surf the Internet. Others stand at the computer, shifting back and forth.

I'm not aware of any studies on the subject of sex and RLS, nor have any been proposed, but I have participated in a number of conversations on the subject, usually late at night with fellow sleepwalkers—in this case also sleeptalkers. Sex works as a diversion but its limitations—having to do with age, enterprise, and energy—are obvious. The sort of sex that one employs for a diversion should be slow-paced. The longer the carnal enterprise, the later the return to the miseries of RLS.

Pets can provide an ideal diversion. Gradually isolated from the rest of her family by the burdens of RLS, Shirley Pourciau of Jarreau, Louisiana, found that her greatest solace was her dog. "I've had a black lab, Medina, for the past five years. She is and has been the best thing that has come into my life. She walks with me when my legs hurt. She licks my legs whenever I stop for a minute, as if to say, I understand. She asks no questions, demands no explanations, doesn't snicker or criticize when I cry or yell in despair. She simply understands."

Some nightwalkers are diverted by cats, though felines are far less likely to follow a nightwalker around, providing the sort of solace conferred by canines in the bleak and especially lonely hours of the early morning.

Dancing and a chiropractor provide some assuagement to Jeanne Pulley of Hopkins, Minnesota: "Since my retirement (I am now seventy-three years old), I found a perfect volunteer job. I joined a group of ladies who dance (tap and jazz) for senior clubs, nursing homes, and schoolchildren. There are fourteen of us; the average age is seventy."

TRAVELING

Traveling, ironically, usually involves a lot of sitting still, and that is a challenge for nightwalkers.

Sitting in an airplane seat for a long flight can be impossible, so nightwalkers use various stratagems to minimize the discomfort. So that she could flex her legs while on an airplane, Pickett Guthrie obtained a letter from the passenger service supervisor of American Airlines. It asks AA employees to let Ms. Guthrie stand up frequently during her flight except for times that may be a threat to her safety—i.e., during turbulence, takeoff, and landing. Another letter to AA from her doctor, which was written in keeping with the spirit of the Americans with Disabilities Act, asked that his patient be assigned an aisle seat, preferably toward the rear of the plane.

Air passengers with RLS should request aisle seats for their own comfort and that of seatmates. The RLS Foundation's Washington liaison, Robert Balkam, advises:

> The Air Carriers Access Act (14 Code of Federal Regulations 382.38) provides that if you identify yourself to an air carrier that assigns seats in advance (not all airlines do) as a passenger with a disability "needing a seat assignment accommodation in order to access and use the carrier's air transportation services," then you will be afforded consideration in your seat assignment. The regulation does not guarantee you an aisle seat. It merely provides the carrier a reason to accommodate your request. . . . Air carriers have a complaint resolution officer, who is supposed to be available by telephone at all times to ticket and gate agents. If you are not satisfied with the response to your seating request, ask the agent to allow you to speak to the carrier's complaint resolution officer.

It will help to have a letter from your physician. The following, written for RLS Foundation board member Sheila Connolly, can serve as a model.

To whom it may concern:

I am writing to ask that flight attendants assigned to planes on the attached itinerary accommodate my patient, _____.

_____ has a neurological disorder called restless legs syndrome, which causes bothersome sensations in the legs, producing an irresistible urge to move. Symptoms are worse when the afflicted individual is at rest, and the physical discomfort, once established, can last for several hours. Symptoms are worse in the evening. Since _____ should avoid sitting longer than 30–45 minutes, the condition is particularly acute during long airplane trips.

In keeping with the spirit of the Americans with Disabilities Act, I request that your attendants make a few simple accommodations that will enable my patient to travel.

1. Please be sure _____ is assigned an aisle seat, preferably in an aisle with more leg room such as the emergency exit aisle or first row.

2. During the flight, please allow her to stand up frequently, perhaps in the galley area or in another place where she will not interfere with food and beverage service or create safety problems.

Thank you in advance for your efforts to accommodate my patient. I hope these precautions will head off the onset of extreme discomfort which, for this patient, can last several hours.

Sincerely, _____, MD

Effective medication is making the lives of nightwalkers much easier, but there are times when one still has to be creative. One man recalls a flight from South Carolina:

Armed with my new medicine, my wife and I were off to London. After boarding I settled in, ordered a drink, and reached for my pill that would ensure a good night's sleep over the Atlantic. As I reached in my kit, I discovered the wrong bottle of pills—simply aspirin. The correct RLS medicine was at home.

Shortly the dancing began and I was pounding on my thighs and stretching like Baryshnikov—to no avail. I got up and started walking. This continued through the night, and as we taxied into the gate, I realized I had done the impossible—walked to England from the United States. Thankfully, my pills were overnighted and I was able to enjoy the rest of the vacation.

Car trips present their own challenges. Professor Elizabeth Tunison describes a family vacation:

I went on a car trip with my son and his family. They chose to go at night so the children would sleep. Before long everyone was asleep, except my son, who was driving, and me. I was in the middle of the backseat with a sleeping child on each side and hundreds of worms crawling inside my legs. I didn't want my son to stop the car for fear it would wake the others. I tried standing on the floor but couldn't, so I put my feet on the backseat, my hands on the back of each front seat, and my back and head against the top. I must have looked like a giant spider or a weird monster, for when my daughter-in-law opened her eyes, she let out a scream that started the children screaming and crying. At least it gave me a chance to get out of the car and walk around for a while.

During a trip to England with my wife and father-in-law, I drove a car with a left-handed manual shift, a right-sided steering wheel, and a right-handed turn signal lever. Neither of my companions wanted to pilot that vehicle, especially since it had to be driven on the left. That coordination test is always a challenge, but this time—shortly after the surgery that made my RLS worse—I drove in a fashion that was bizarre and certainly dangerous.

Every five minutes or so I had to find a place to turn off, stop, leap out, and walk. Back in the car, I edged uneasily into traffic, beginning soon thereafter to search for another place to exit. My passengers tried to express compassion, but I could tell that they were mainly worried for their lives. Sensing that, I became even more tense and twitchy, and my course more treacherous. I now realize that at the time I was not dealing constructively with the reality of RLS.

In contrast, Bob Guthrie, husband of Pickett Guthrie, an RLS Foundation cofounder, came up with the solution of building a stationary exercise bicycle in their van. Pickett, whose RLS was so severe that she couldn't sit still for more than a few minutes in the passenger seat, was thereby able to move her legs—by pedaling—as he drove. They were again able to take trips.

FAMILY AND FRIENDS

No one has done more in efforts to vanquish RLS than Robert H. Waterman Jr., former chairman of the RLS Foundation board of directors, yet he recalls being plagued for most of his life with the phrase, "It's just in your head":

The utterance comes from all quarters. Doctors, who above all ought to know better, have dismissed my complaints with this simple phrase. Well-meaning friends and colleagues have told me this with some regularity. My dad made it clear to mom, my sister, and me that he certainly considered our common disease a matter of our collectively addled craniums. Even my wife thought the disease "psychosomatic" for the first fifteen years of our marriage.

It's too bad there isn't a pill that could produce RLS symptoms in disbelievers. A pill that lasted for two or three days would be enough. A physical therapist told me that she had once taken a medicine (probably an antidepressant) that did cause RLS. "It went on all night long!" she exclaimed, the memory still vivid. "I thought I'd go nuts! I can't imagine having to go through a second night." She now recognizes the disease in her patients and, having obtained information from the RLS Foundation, can provide helpful advice.

Educating others is an essential part of coping successfully with RLS. Dr. Daniel Picchietti points out that while we can't duplicate the problematic pulling sensation, it is possible to describe the consequences of sleep deprivation:

> Nearly everyone, especially medical personnel, has gone through periods when they are severely sleep deprived and can remember how hard it was to function. Your mind runs a little slower, you become irritable, little things bother you, you feel sluggish, perhaps depressed. Every task seems like climbing a mountain. Imagine what it would be like to be that way *all the time.*

Some nightwalkers are also daytime sufferers, which limits social life even more than sleep deprivation. Barbara Diamon of Diamond Bar, California, has reported that she often refused invitations because "it is too embarrassing to be seen standing and wiggling."

Juanita Therrell of Bellevue, Washington, couldn't get relief during the day as her doctor was not willing to prescribe anything for her severe daytime symptoms. The simplest routines of home life were disrupted. "I could not stand still in the kitchen to prepare dinner. I left cooking for my husband to finish while I went outside and walked. I ate dinner while pacing the floor in total agony." Fortunately, Juanita has since found another doctor and another medication that has allowed her to function during the day again. After twenty-six years of interrupted sleep, she now is able to stay in bed at night.

About half of American marriages end in divorce. One cause of marital distress, along with financial irritants, confused communications, and sexual disharmony, is, yes, RLS. One might think of snoring, sleep apnea, and the use of sleeping medications as a greater threat to wedded peace, but according to the National Sleep Foundation's 2005 Sleep in America poll, they don't matter, matrimonially speaking. RLS does.[2]

The study showed that RLS symptoms affected 14 percent of women and 11 percent of men "a few nights a week or more." Two causes of marital strain among those tormented couples were leg movement during sleep (in PLM)—kicking the bedmate—and frequent awakenings (in RLS) that made sharing a bed or even a bedroom impractical. Add to that source of tension the effect on a family's social life of a person who can't sit through a movie, play, concert, lecture, or even a meal, and you have a significant challenge for any relationship. According to Dr. Richard Allen, one-third of RLS patients report that they wake the person they sleep with an average of three times per month, and nearly one-tenth of these people report that they no longer sleep in the same bed with their partner.[3]

"My husband has RLS and it has been pure hell for us," wrote Michele Crandell of Melrose, Wisconsin. "He gets it so bad, sometimes he'll look at me dead on his feet, wanting to sleep so much that he has a complete and utter look of misery and despair on his face. We cannot sleep together and I feel totally impotent as his helpmate because I cannot help him."

Margarette Fuhr observes that RLS is easier to cope with when the family understands that it is a disease: no one is to blame.

> My husband has been a dear friend through this disease. My RLS has not been easy for him, and at first, when symptoms worsened, I think he found it and me very difficult to live with. Slowly but surely as we both became more educated about the syndrome, and as he saw me truly suffering, he understood that it was not my fault. He has supported me in innumerable ways, both physically and in my heart. He plans shorter days on car trips so that the medication will not wear off and have me climbing from front to backseat and back again, which I have done. These shorter days are hard on a German who likes a schedule that gets us there on time. He patiently finishes meals alone while I am forced to walk around. He often sits alone in the theater while I stand in the back.

It is unusual in marriages, but William H. Amos of Lyndonville, Vermont, was pleased to discover that he was wrong and his wife was right: "Hallelujah! For years my wife has accused me of kicking her in bed at short intervals while I'm fast asleep—and I've stoutly denied it." Now, thanks to learning about RLS, "I am enlightened and my wife is vindicated. I guess I *have* been kicking her all these years."

Buzzy Katz of Sarasota, Florida, recalled that his late wife, Ruth, had a heart condition, diabetes, emphysema, and RLS. Of all the things wrong with her, Ruth felt the worst was the restless legs. Many nights they would spend together in the kitchen—she standing up and doing the crossword puzzles that she so enjoyed, and he standing behind her, holding her up. Ruth would be so tired that she'd be ready to collapse, but she just couldn't sleep because of the legs.

> We would stand there for a while and then I would get her to walk around the house a little bit and I would hold her—around the house, around the house. And finally, maybe three or four o'clock in the morning, it would let up, we'd get into bed and finally get some sleep. It was a terrible period.
>
> One time I caught her, she was trying to get her medications, they were in a very high place where she couldn't reach them. And I happened to hear her and I came in the kitchen; she had gotten a chair and she was climbing up in the chair to reach the medications. And she had just reached the point because of the restless legs. She was going to do herself in. She had never, never considered anything like that with all the problems she went through, but the restless legs just got to her. You know, with all her sicknesses, all her ailments, and all her suffering, she had a wonderful sense of humor. We always joked; she poked fun at herself. But she could not poke fun at restless legs.

Jealousy of the unaffected mate is not unusual. Faye Litman of Mound, Minnesota, described how:

> I listen with envy, and occasional guilty hostility, to my husband quietly snoring in the bedroom across the hall, undisturbed by the movement or noises I create in our small house. How I have always coveted his peaceful, sleep-filled nights, oblivious to sick, hungry, or

bad-dreaming children years ago, a noisy ill-functioning furnace or refrigerator, history-making storms, flapping house parts in strong winds, a dog or a cat restless because of unusual activity outside. . . .

My life now is not what I thought it would be. I planned to work well into my sixties, travel, entertain friends, enjoy theater, orchestra, and movies. I watch movies and travel videos while pacing at home. I seek out early-afternoon activity after getting jump-started and mostly free of medicine hangover by mid to late morning. I'm not dependable; plans will change depending upon what kind of night I've had. By 5 p.m. I am already a restless, cranky, tired body.

My husband moves in his own world—helpful, but mystified and uncomprehending of what my life is really like now. It isn't other people's fault that they don't get it. They could help by *not* offering advice and instead just saying, "I'm sorry life is like this for you now. We'll work around it."

If some adults have to struggle to explain RLS to a doctor, it's obvious that they are faced with a tough task when trying to help a child understand the disease. It may be best not to try for anyone under four. A parent will probably try to compare the sensations to those of legs going to sleep. But if that's a feeling most children would recognize, it's not one that is easy to demonstrate. In the search for sympathy, one can legitimately explain the agony of RLS with friends. But an attempt to demonstrate lower limb distress to one's younger offspring would alarm them and embarrass you.

Dating presents its own special problems. "Although I had trouble with my legs as a child," one woman recalls, "my first memory of being miserable was on a date. I spent the entire time in the lobby and restroom of a movie theater while my date watched the show. That was someone I had wanted to date for a long time, and needless to say it was my first and last date with him."

CHAPTER 8

Special Challenges

Avoid fried meats which angry up the blood. If your stomach
disputes you, lie down and pacify it with cool thoughts. Keep the
juices flowing by jangling around gently as you move. Go very
light on the vices, such as carrying on in society. The social
ramble ain't restful. Avoid running at all times. Don't look back.
Something might be gaining on you.

—Leroy (Satchel) Paige, "How to Stay Young"

THE ROLE OF STRESS

When stress meets RLS, stress worsens RLS, which worsens
stress, which worsens RLS, which . . .

According to the Society for Neuroscience, more than half of
all Americans feel "a great deal of stress" at least once a week.[1] Most
of us are under some stress as part of our daily lives, and occasionally under a lot of stress triggered by money problems, domestic
disputes, looming deadlines, overwork, a letter from the IRS, or a
cab ride in New York City. Stress can be beneficial—it may increase
one's speed when being pursued by a lion, for example—but such
occasions are rare.

Numerous ailments are aggravated by stress—ulcers, headaches, heart trouble, acne, back pain, chronic fatigue, gastrointestinal distress, and asthma, to name but a few. Since stress can cause some diseases and can aggravate many, it's hardly surprising that sleep experts believe that while stress can't cause RLS, it certainly can exacerbate it and thereby worsen sleep deprivation. And sleep deprivation, according to researchers like Stanford University geneticist Neil Risch, can weaken the immune system. So in theory at least, the immune systems of RLS victims are weakened by stress. This may be a particular problem for those whose immune systems are already weakened by advancing age—the same inexorable process that often worsens their RLS.

In an interview with the author, Dr. Bruce Ehrenberg points out that RLS "would be an exceptional disease if there were no psychological component, involving, as it does, both sensory and motor disorders." Given the role of the neurotransmitter dopamine in RLS, and given the way stress can alter the complex interplay of neurotransmitters, it's likely that RLS is to some degree affected by brain chemical events. "Sleep deprivation of any cause will affect the efficiency of immune functions. Therefore, all causes of mortality relating to immune responses, including cancer, may be elevated in those with severe sleep deprivation." In his chapter "Sleep, Longevity, and the Immune System" in *The Promise of Sleep*, Dr. William Dement lists studies that seem to confirm that "from the perspective of longevity, sleep may turn out to be more important than most people think." None of those studies prove a causal relationship between amount of sleep and life span, "but the results are extremely suggestive."

There is a great deal of anecdotal evidence of an RLS-stress connection. My mother was convinced, after decades of experience, that anxiety could make her RLS worse. As my own symptoms intensified, I came to the same conclusion, as have many other nightwalkers.

But we must be careful. It is possible that a stressful day, or the prospect of one—or, ironically, even a medicine taken to avoid stress or its consequences—could cause insomnia. And insomnia would, of course, make RLS victims more aware of their disagreeable sensations. Still, it seems reasonable to assume that RLS, sleep deprivation, and stress can all reinforce each other.

Prudence would dictate, therefore, that those of us who are tortured by RLS act on the assumption that stress, for whatever reason, is an ally of our enemy. Accordingly, it would be wise to follow the advice of experts on ways of reducing stress and improving sleep. (See Chapter 4.)

RLS victims may want to try diversions that will keep stressful thoughts at a distance. While walking around the room or marching in place, listen to a soporific audio book or peaceful music on a tape or CD, or watch a sport in which you have little interest. There is widespread agreement in the health community that having someone to talk to is also a good way to reduce stress. That's one reason why joining a support group can help stressed-out RLS victims.

One should, of course, try to abolish the causes of stress, but we all know how difficult that is. The more immediate goal should be to find medication designed to moderate RLS symptoms. With the aid of an informed physician, the wise nightwalker will concentrate on the main enemy—the disorder that causes those stress-inducing symptoms.

WHEN RLS BECOMES LIFE-THREATENING

Nightwalkers who have not found adequate support often feel forsaken, abandoned by those who don't understand. They suffer loneliness, weariness, fits of crying, and despair. Some think about amputating the offending limbs. I've heard of two women who stabbed their legs, one with a knife, the other with scissors. It is common for nightwalkers who suffer from other serious ailments to assert that RLS is by far the worst. As one woman has reported, "I have breast cancer, aplastic anemia, glaucoma, high blood pressure, and a few other odds and ends—and all of them together are nothing compared to RLS."

The discomfort is hard enough on the psyche, especially when the arms and upper torso are involved, but it's the sleep deprivation that can push sufferers into a suicidal state. It is not surprising that a recent study of over three thousand people in Turkey found that people with RLS were more likely than others to experience anxiety and depression.[2] Some RLS victims—no one knows how many—actually choose suicide.

Dr. Philip Becker, of the Sleep Medicine Institute, describes the danger:

Since RLS is often a lifelong and potentially severe disorder, it can leave the nightwalker feeling discouraged, fatigued, and burdened. Dread for another next night of suffering can cause hopelessness and heightened anxiety. In predisposed individuals, depression may develop. As depression deepens into a clinical disorder, thoughts of suicide may intrude. The wish for release from the suffering of RLS may become a preoccupation. Any person with RLS, or the loved ones, must then recognize that it is time to seek professional help for the cloud of hopelessness and depression.

The thought of suicide often crossed my bedeviled mind. Such dark thoughts reached their peak one horrific night while I was on a cruise in the middle of a storm in the Bay of Biscay. The storm was so severe that nearly all the passengers were seasick, including the ship's doctor and me. Because the ship was storm-tossed, I couldn't walk. Because I had RLS, I couldn't lie down. Because I was violently seasick, I couldn't keep my medicine, or anything else, in my stomach. As anyone who has had it knows, seasickness alone can make one feel suicidal. So can severe RLS. Combined, the two made me seriously consider hurling myself into the angry sea. Meanwhile, to add insult to injury, my wife, Alice, a seasoned sailor who doesn't get seasick, was asleep—and, as usual, smiling.

One desperate man in Michigan reported that he "walked for two weeks straight, fourteen nights, and didn't sleep a wink. Then I tried to commit suicide by stabbing myself in the stomach." Leona Meyer, of Monango, North Dakota, confessed, "If I were thinking only of myself, I would have ended this misery long since. On one of my visits with my doctor he said, 'Leona, I just don't have anything more that I can give you.' I offhandedly remarked that I guessed maybe the next referral I'd be asking him for was Dr. Kevorkian. He answered, 'I wouldn't blame you.' I'm sure that one reason RLS has not been given much priority is that it is not a life-threatening condition. If it can drive you to suicide, it is definitely life-threatening."

Helen Keith, of Mariposa, California, recognizes that her life has been saved by medication. "My father had this and killed himself at age forty-nine because he could get no rest. At least I can go on with my life."

Many nightwalkers have reported brushes with death, like the one described by Kenneth Humphreys, of Newport, Tennessee: "I went to a hardware store to get a .357 magnum pistol. The clerk said I could have it if I signed a paper for the sheriff and chief of police. I thought a person on crutches and barely getting around would be so obvious, I decided to forget the idea. Then I began to think I could drive off a bridge . . ."

"I almost shot myself in the leg," a man in New York reported, "thinking if I damaged something, it might stop. I am going out of my mind." Without appropriate treatment, many nightwalkers end up fearing for their sanity. One woman reported that after two months of severe sleep deprivation, "I became slightly psychotic, my driving became erratic and dangerous, my memory and concentration poor, I was depressed and felt like I was falling apart. It is difficult to make commitments when you don't know which days you are going to be a total zombie from lack of sleep, so you wind up with no life at all. . . . Death, for me at least, would be preferable."

Thoughts of self-mutilation may plague nightwalkers who remain untreated. One woman "begged my husband to cut my legs off with a buzz saw so I could get some sleep. And at times I think he was tempted. My constant movement in bed kept him awake—and irritated him—until we recently found out that I wasn't making this up."

When one considers self-injury or suicide, as I have, it doesn't necessarily mean that one is close to doing it. Presumably, even among the most severely afflicted nightwalkers, only a tiny minority actually try to leave life. But those who do choose permanent slumber over sleeplessness provide proof that RLS can be a dire and even deadly disease.

Suicidal thoughts aren't an inevitable product of severe RLS, but it's wise to devise a tactic for dealing with them. The chapter on sleep lists several diversions. Try all of them. Employ humor, especially the sort—whether in a book or movie or TV sitcom—that involves absurdities. My recommendation would be anything by P. G. Wodehouse, Dave Barry, or Carl Hiaasen.

My further advice to the seriously afflicted is to get in touch with others in a similar state. That will be easier if you belong to a support group, of course; if you don't, start one.

I assume that you will be sharing your travails with your doctor. His role should be to offer different treatments when others have failed. If you are fortunate he or she will be a voice of reason, compassion, and encouragement.

SOCIETAL COSTS

What do the grounding of the *Exxon Valdez,* the near meltdown at Three Mile Island, the Bhopal chemical catastrophe, and the explosion of the space shuttle *Challenger* have in common? According to Dr. William Dement, they were all caused totally or in part by sleepy people.

Sleep deprivation, often a major component of RLS, can lead to depression, irritability, and fatigue—all of which make day-to-day living a challenge. The National Institutes of Health summarizes the consequences of restless legs syndrome:

Direct results of RLS include discomfort, sleep disturbances, and fatigue. These consequences have a secondary impact on functioning by affecting occupational activities, social activities, and family life.

Disrupted sleep and an inability to tolerate sedentary activities can lead to job loss, a compromised ability to enjoy life, and problems with relationships.[3]

Clearly, RLS costs more than lives. It is impossible to determine the exact monetary costs of RLS: there are too many variables, and figures on sleep costs in general don't always agree, since it isn't easy to conduct precise studies on the subject of sleep. For example, there is no way to calculate the debilitating effects of RLS on other diseases. Serious ailments like heart disease and cancer can be worsened by RLS.

Official reports on the cause of accidents can foil researchers. (Who knows whether sleep deprivation was as much the cause of an accident as booze?) Vague answers to survey questions can warp results ("I think that I slept only a couple of hours that night, but I'm not sure"), as can questions requiring subjective replies ("Do you have trouble sleeping?").

While precise RLS cost calculations are elusive, this much is clear: enormous penalties are paid by everyone in society for the ignorance and indifference that attend the broader subject of sleep deprivation.

One estimate places the total annual cost of sleep disorders at $45 billion, including $18 billion of lost productivity, $14 billion in health care costs, and $13 billion in costs of motor vehicle accidents caused by sleep deprivation.[4]

Again, according to the National Commission on Sleep Disorders Research (NCSDR), direct and indirect economic losses every year as a result of all untreated sleep disorders and sleep deprivation are in the tens of billions of dollars. *Direct* costs to the nation's health care bill—the cost of sleep disorders and sleep deprivation—are estimated at \$15.8 billion by the NCSDR.[5] There is no way to determine what portion of those huge sums is attributable to RLS.

Some medications taken by RLS patients carry a warning that the substance can cause "sleep attacks"—sudden loss of consciousness. Such attacks are fortunately very rare. (It should be noted here that no evidence shows that RLS victims suffer from *excessive* daytime somnolence, or that they cause more road accidents than others.)

I used to dictate into a recorder while driving, and on more than one occasion, after I'd been walking all night, my assistant heard me slipping into sleep. Words on the tape became slurred and increasingly meaningless. That practice was stupid, of course, and I've given it up, but at the time I could easily have become one of the sleepy drivers who cause more than 100,000 car accidents a year in the United States, more than 40,000 of which result in injuries, 1,500 in death. The American Medical Association arrived at these figures after reviewing more than ninety studies on traffic accidents and sleep deprivation.[6] The same study concluded that 13 percent of automobile deaths are caused by people who fall asleep at the wheel.

A survey of 1,000 New York State drivers revealed that 26 percent of them reported falling asleep at the wheel in the previous year.[7] (That figure would be somewhat higher if it included drivers who perished while asleep.) People who suffer from daytime RLS are at risk not only because of fatigue, but because they are forced, while driving, to stretch their legs constantly—a practice that has not, as far as I know, been included in any safety studies but one that, I can testify, can result in erratic, perilous performance on the highways.

RLS can contribute to other kinds of accidents. The husband of a member of the Southern California support group wrote to the RLS Foundation:

> I regret to inform you of the death of my beloved wife of fifty years. . . . While warming her restless legs in front of the fireplace a week ago, she had a slight stroke, which apparently caused her to roll too close to the fire, and caught her clothes on fire. That resulted in second- and third-degree burns over 60 percent of her body. After homograft surgery, she suffered a major stroke, and there was no medical remedy.

He asked friends in lieu of flowers to contribute to the RLSF to further research into RLS, to find the cause and a real cure.

Accidents are only one of the challenges that RLS presents in the workplace. It is impossible to know how many people have lost their jobs, or failed to advance in them, because of RLS. This, however, is certain: anyone who has a severe case of RLS will be unable to work as efficiently as someone who gets enough sleep. Those who, because of sleep deprivation, stagger around during the day are likely to attract the attention of fellow employees or customers. That would be especially true, one hopes, of sleep-deprived pilots, air traffic controllers, and brain surgeons. (It's a sobering thought, but it is virtually certain that *some* air traffic controllers, pilots, and brain surgeons are among the perhaps 15 percent of the population that has RLS.) Augmentation, which pushes symptoms into daytime, can create problems for workers as well.

A veterinarian from San Mateo, California, had such a severe case of RLS that he considered giving up his practice. He couldn't remain in one position long enough to treat his sometimes equally restless patients. Unable to sleep much at night, he was drowsy all day. His social life was also affected. He would sit down, fall asleep for a couple of minutes, awaken, stand up to pace and flex his legs, sit down, fall asleep, and so on. His professional and social existence was restored after he saw a neurologist who referred him to the Stanford University Sleep Research Center, where he was successfully treated. The treatment, he said, "miraculously gave me back my life."

Without effective treatment, nightwalkers in the past have lost jobs or been seriously handicapped in their performance, because of RLS. A nurse in Minnesota recalled how her symptoms forced her to retire at the age of fifty-five. "I felt so incompetent, became very anxious, and my body hurt after a shift at the hospital. All because of lack of sleep and rest. My job became physically and mentally exhausting and was taking its toll on my body and life."

"I had a great job as vice president of marketing for a large Midwest defense electronics company," wrote Charles Skillas, of Norcross, Georgia, in the midnineties:

I started there in 1968. I had my first RLS experience in 1970. At the time it was just an annoyance, but it rapidly grew into a debilitating condition.

I tried several doctors who put me on various medications. By 1974 I was experiencing extreme sleep deprivation and also suffering from the side effects of the medicines. I was constantly getting addicted and had to go through withdrawal so the drugs would work again to let me sleep.

Meanwhile, I was experiencing great difficulty at my job. I was working on two to three hours of sleep and suffering the hangover effects of the heavy medications.

A neurologist told me it was an emotional problem and that I should see a psychiatrist. I actually spent five weeks in the Neuropsychiatric Research Institute at the University of Michigan, during which time they gave me very potent drugs for depression because they thought the RLS was from depression.

After leaving the hospital I went to a new neurologist, who said I had RLS. *This was the first time it was diagnosed correctly.* The neurologist gave me Dilantin, which I couldn't take because it made my gums bleed. So back to the barbiturates. Actually now they put me on Xanax, a benzodiazepine drug that was terribly addictive, which I didn't know.

By this time I could no longer work. I quit my job and moved to Atlanta. In 1991 I had to go to the detox unit to get off Xanax. I could hardly function. I now began to think of suicide. In the meantime the doctors I went to continued to prescribe the same heavy drugs. It was fifteen months before I could begin to function and get a job.

I have gone as much as six days without sleep. One becomes on the verge of psychotic, so you must then go back to the drugs and get some sleep. As you can see, the RLS has deeply affected my life for twenty-five years. Fortunately, the drugs I am now taking work fairly well and I am able to get enough sleep so that I can function.

RLS can take an enormous toll on productivity. Over the years many nightwalkers have had to sell their businesses or take early retirement. In some cases the side effects of the drugs taken to treat symptoms have made work impossible. A retired hospital laboratory supervisor recalled:

By 1975 I was working sixteen hours a day and sleeping about two. This problem began to control me. One day I was talking to a technician and I had a quick blackout and noticed the technician looking very puzzled at me, and he said, "Ken, what just happened to you?" I had gone to sleep standing up. At night I often fell out of bed. Things continued to get worse and I never got any rest. I worked at my job and then I was building a house on a farm I purchased. The pressure was so great I began to break down. I had to retire.

Over the years such workplace problems have afflicted thousands of RLS sufferers. The loss of a job can have devastating financial and psychological consequences. It's sad to think of all the people who might have kept their jobs had their efforts to find a treatment been rewarded. It's especially sad to think of those who didn't even know the name of the disease that deprived them of their livelihood.

THE CHALLENGE FOR NURSING HOMES

Stress takes on new meaning when applied to RLS patients suffering in nursing homes. Indeed, I was motivated to write this book in part by the suffering in such institutions caused by RLS and PLM. Since both diseases disproportionately affect the elderly, it seemed obvious that nursing homes would be sites of intense nightly anguish. My assumption was corroborated by Dr. Richard Allen, director of the Sleep Disorders Center at Johns Hopkins University and former chair of the RLS Foundation Medical Advisory Board: "All our studies indicate that as many as 10 percent of people in nursing homes have RLS, but nothing like that number are being diagnosed. Tens of thousands are being missed, apparently, *and many are in serious trouble.*" Further, no one has exact figures, but Dr. Allen believes that there are at least 9 million elderly living at home (who may or may not have skilled health care), and that it is reasonable to assume that a million of those elderly are afflicted to some degree with RLS and PLM.

In the year 2000, the federal government imposed fines on one thousand of the nation's seventeen thousand nursing homes. The fines were for substandard care, which, according to a report sent to Congress earlier that year, was largely caused by understaffing.[8] A shortage of nurses and nurse's aides contributed to an increase in the incidence of severe bedsores, malnutrition, and abnormal weight loss. Many patients end up hospitalized for life-threatening infections, dehydration, congestive heart failure, and other preventable or treatable afflictions. In such institutions, what are the odds that RLS and PLM will be identified and treated? The answer is that thousands of patients are tormented every night.

Some doctors are dismissive with the elderly. They may be bored by the plethora of aches and pains, often of uncertain provenance, that accompany advancing age; others are frustrated by patients who have a hard time describing their ailments. A doctor with such an attitude is unlikely to pay attention to a patient who complains of sleeplessness caused by a creepy-crawly sensation. In an ideal world, such doctors wouldn't practice in nursing homes, but the world inhabited by the aged is far from ideal.

Not all RLS victims in nursing homes experience the deep depression or intense anxiety that the ailment can cause, but many do. And if their disease is undiagnosed and untreated, the odds are that they are living in despair—bewildered, groggy with fatigue, and perhaps prevented from walking at night, which their legs demand. Living under such conditions creates stress, which, as we have seen, weakens the immune system and makes a population already vulnerable to disease even more vulnerable.

Other illnesses among this population are exacerbated by RLS and PLM. As we have seen, some people suffering from cancer, heart disease, or other debilitating conditions say that RLS is the worst because it won't let them sleep and relief is transitory. What irony, then, that many elderly patients are being treated for everything except the ailment that makes everything else worse and that, therefore, causes them the greatest misery.

Try to put yourself in the slippers of an aged man or woman (more likely to be the latter because women live longer) in a nursing home, who struggles, night after ghastly night, to get out of bed so that she can pace the halls, or at least her room, and who is prevented from doing so by aides, nurses, and doctors who haven't an inkling of the agony they are imposing on her. Only then would you fully understand how much unnecessary pain is inflicted on the innocent by the ignorant.

John W. Cresnicki, of Frankfurt, Michigan, wrote about his mother, a ninety-six-year-old with RLS:

> We have been to numerous doctors who examined her and stated that nothing was wrong with her. [Some say] that she naps too much in the daytime and that causes her to imagine that she is not able to sleep at night. [But] my mother, whose mind is sharp for her age, insists that her legs are the cause. . . . Right now she is in a nursing home and still suffering from this affliction. My wife (who is a nurse) keeps telling the nursing home of her condition, but the doctor and nurse who attend her think we are worrywarts and they don't do a thing.

Similarly, a woman from Brookfield, Wisconsin, described her husband's aunt, who was eighty-seven and always complaining of RLS symptoms. The doctors said it was her age and hinted that she was demented, although in fact she was sharp and quick-witted.

In an interview, Dr. J. Steven Poceta, of the Scripps Clinic and Research Foundation, pointed out that some nursing home occupants, "confined to bed because of a stroke or a broken bone or some disease that causes confusion, suffer as much as those who have been restrained. These conditions tend to cause akathisia, a feeling of restlessness that you can have all over your body—restlessness that is quite similar to RLS. Some nursing homes also use antidepressants, like Prozac, which also worsen PLM and, apparently, RLS."

It is urgent that nursing home staff and other health care workers be educated about RLS. The good news is that identifying RLS is not rocket science, and training takes only an hour or two. Nurses, who can play pivotal roles in getting relief for their patients, have became the object of awareness campaigns. Once trained to identify the disease, nurses and health aides can help victims by providing them with opportunities to walk and move their limbs.

Restraints have long been used in nursing homes, and for just as long restricting their use has been a goal of nursing home reform. There are some instances in which the use of restraints is justified, but those cases are greatly outnumbered by examples of abuse, of restraints used to punish or as a substitute for nursing care in an understaffed institution. Far fewer restraints would be required for the elderly if medications appropriate to RLS patients were used by health care providers in nursing homes.

If you are faced with the tough task of choosing a nursing home, either for yourself or for a relative or friend, you will want to ask a lot of questions. If the prospective resident is a nightwalker, find out whether the doctors, nurses, and aides are familiar with RLS and PLM. If answers to questions on that subject aren't reassuring, keep looking. With effort and attention, RLS in the elderly can be managed in a humane way and needless suffering prevented.

Another question posed to nursing home officials is, "Does the Americans with Disabilities Act cover RLS victims?" The answer points out that it's the disabilities that are spelled out by the law—not the disorders. So some of the disabilities that can arise from having RLS can be covered. For instance, people do get accommodations on airplanes as a valid medical condition. A valid medical condition related to RLS may also be covered by Social Security disability. Many health insurance plans do cover RLS.

DEPRESSION

It isn't surprising to discover that about 40 percent of adults with RLS describe symptoms that resemble depression. These include depressed mood, diminished interests, feelings of worthlessness, thoughts of death, weight gain or loss, insomnia or excessive sleepiness, fatigue or loss of energy, diminished concentration, mental/physical sluggishness, or agitation.

A pamphlet published by the RLS Foundation entitled *Special Considerations in Treating Depression* is helpful when trying to sort out symptoms, syndromes, and treatments.

The consensus among experts is that the first step for a depressed RLS patient should be to assess the severity of the depression-related symptoms. If the conclusion is that poor sleep is probably the villain, it is best to deal with that sleep disorder first. It will then be easier to measure the severity and nature of the depression.

I can testify that anyone burdened by the mental fatigue accompanying severe RLS is unlikely to be in shape for successful self-analysis or a profitable program with a psychiatrist.

CHAPTER 9

Hope

Attempt the end, and never stand to doubt;
Nothing's so hard but search will find it out.

—ROBERT HERRICK, "SEEK AND FIND"

EARLY RESEARCH

The British neurologist Sir Thomas Willis was the first physician to describe RLS and PLM, in his *London Practice of Physick* in 1683 (originally written in Latin). Willis was also the first to report that the condition could be treated with an opiatelike medication that was similar to some now in use. RLS symptoms may have been more common in the seventeenth century because of the medical practice of bloodletting, which lowered a patient's iron levels.

Almost nothing was added to knowledge of RLS for nearly three centuries. Most doctors who observed symptoms in the eighteenth and nineteenth centuries identified the disease as "hysterical," a sign of mental stress. The condition became known as *anxietas tibiarum*, or "anxious legs." In 1861 a German neurologist observed that "it really is as if a spirit of restlessness and compulsion to move has invaded the legs of the afflicted person. Every moment sees the legs brought into a different position: drawn up, stretched out, abducted, spread apart, and crossed over one another."[1]

In 1913 R. Bing described "a form of bone paraesthesia" as "a dull feeling, difficult to define, in the shin bones." He also identified this condition as anxietas tibiarum. But he then went on to depict "a corresponding feeling experienced in healthy persons," whom he distinguished from the presumably deranged victims of anxietas tibiarum. Healthy persons, Bing wrote, refer to the onset of the disease as "when my legs became panic stricken."[2]

Although in the late nineteenth century neurologists began to note that the affliction was familial, they continued to report it as a form of neurosis—or "anxious legs"—until the 1940s. As is still true today, the clinical studies that brought RLS out of the "it's a form of hysteria" era and into the light of modern medicine were conducted by researchers in several countries, especially England, France, Italy, Germany, Sweden, Canada, and the United States.

The first neurologist to report that RLS was a physical, not psychological disorder was H. Oppenheim in 1923. After describing the symptoms, the German doctor wrote, "It can become an agonizing torture, lasting for years or decades and can be passed on to, and occur in, other members of the family."[3]

Giant strides toward the understanding of RLS and PLM were made in the 1940s. In the first year of that decade, J. D. Mussio-Fournier and F. Rawak described the clinical features of RLS and, in so doing, provided more evidence that it was not a psychiatric disease. They correctly believed it was a disorder of the central nervous system. They also concluded that the ailment could be transmitted genetically and that it appeared with unexpected frequency during pregnancy.[4]

Realizing, with further research, that the upper limbs could also be involved, the French scientists named the disease *agitation paresthesique des extrémités,* or paresthetic restlessness of the extremities. F. G. Allison, a Canadian doctor who suffered from RLS himself, described the disease in 1943 and wrote the first description of the associated syndrome now known as PLM.[5] "Leg jitters" is how Allison described the rhythmic involuntary muscular jerks that characterize PLM. Other researchers labeled that syndrome nocturnal myoclonus (*myo* = muscle; *clonic* = jerks), a name that was used for several years to describe PLM.

The importance of Karl A. Ekbom's pioneering work is reflected by the use in Europe of "Ekbom's syndrome" to describe RLS—and by repeated references to his work in medical literature. Ekbom's monographs, based on more extensive clinical studies than had been conducted by any of his predecessors, showed the effectiveness of sedating drugs and confirmed several associated causes of the disease like pregnancy, genetics, and iron deficiency.

He believed the prevalence of the disease to be about 11 percent—a figure akin to those emerging from recent studies. Although, contrary to Ekbom's belief, poor circulation in the legs is no longer considered to be a major cause of the disorder, many researchers think that vascular disease may play a role in some cases. Dr. Sonia Ancoli-Israel showed that behavioral techniques that increase blood flow in the legs provide relief for some patients.[6]

Enlightened by the work of Dr. Ekbom, Dr. C. P. Symonds, who first used the phrase *nocturnal myoclonus* in 1953 to describe what was eventually known as PLM, with Dr. Elio Lugaresi and their colleagues at the University of Bologna, made the next significant advance.[7] Employing nighttime recording instruments, Dr. Lugaresi discovered that many people who had RLS also had PLM. News about RLS traveled slowly back then. Dr. Lugaresi observed, "When we first encountered a case of RLS in 1962, we found ourselves, like many neurologists and virtually all general practitioners, wholly unaware of the existence of this syndrome."[8]

The American clinical researcher Arthur Walters was primarily responsible for the formation, in 1993, of the International RLS Study Group, which a year later proposed and published a definition for the diagnosis of RLS.[9]

The work of Ekbom, Lugaresi, and others provided a foundation for late twentieth and early twenty-first-century researchers. Since most medications that work for PLM also work for RLS, and since PLM twitches can easily be recorded, researchers were able to identify medications that worked for RLS by trying them on patients with PLM.

WHERE WE ARE TODAY

Although we have only a rudimentary understanding of the causes of RLS, the preponderance of information supports classifying the condition as a "disorder of sensorimotor integration." Movement-disorder specialists, as well as geneticists, today perform much of the RLS research.

They still face a tortuous task. Impressive progress has been made in laboratories since the 1940s, but researchers remain handicapped by a lack of funds, the paucity of earlier studies upon which to build, and the difficulty of identifying and measuring the disease.

Here are some of the hurdles ahead.

As we saw in the discussion of dopamine, much remains to be learned about its pathways and functions, as well as about the role of other neurotransmitters and other brain functions.

In addition, it is hard to measure RLS. Using recordings during sleep, it is fairly easy to identify and measure PLM, but no scientific instruments are helpful in the identification of RLS. (True, electromyography—EMG—can be used to measure tibial muscle movement, and actigraphs record limb activity. But their significance may be compromised by subjective studies in which RLS is mimicked by, for example, diabetic polyneuropathy with nighttime paresthesias.)

It is possible to confirm changes in brain iron of RLS victims, but only by fairly special tests, such as a brain-imaging study done with magnetic resonance imaging (MRI). Even more accurate studies can be done by examining tissue from people who have donated their brains after death—tissue available to researchers at the RLS Foundation collection at the Harvard Brain Tissue Resource Center. Maintaining this facility and paying for the research is very expensive, but foundation board members, RLS victims themselves, realizing that such a resource could be the source of scientific breakthroughs, established this facility in 2000.

Researchers have been handicapped by a lack of funds. Until the RLS Foundation was formed in 1992, there was no place to promote awareness of RLS or to raise money for research projects. The medical community, like the pharmaceutical industry, was largely ignorant of the disease. Only recently has the National Institutes of Health, the primary source for investigator-initiated biomedical research funding, begun to award grants to those studying RLS. The RLS Foundation now provides "seed funds" to several projects each year, hoping to kick-start research on RLS that can go on to find federal funding. This has already happened with several research projects.

(Researchers themselves should do more to familiarize colleagues with RLS. One effective technique: at scientific conferences, ask victims to describe the affliction and answer questions about it. I participated in seminars of this sort and was impressed by the large number of physicians who came up afterward to say that they had previously had no idea of how grievous the disease could be.)

Some research funds have been provided recently by pharmaceutical companies. Those grants, understandably, usually involve prevalence studies and the development of medications that promise to profit sponsoring companies. As a result, behavior, nutrition, and other nondrug therapies are largely ignored.

Limited funds dictate limited trials. Studies have been largely short-term single-drug trials, often limited to small numbers of patients. Long-term large-scale studies, involving comparisons of different drugs and alternative therapies, are urgently needed. Researchers are also eager to conduct long-term studies of drug risks and benefits.

With the new century came welcome interest in RLS by various institutes of the NIH. Supporting research with the RLS Foundation came mainly from the National Institute of Neurological Disorders and Stroke, although other institutes were involved in the 1999 conference called The Dopamine Connection. Participants agreed that one likely cause of RLS is impaired transmission of that vital neurotransmitter. This led them to conclude that further research should include the development of an animal model; additional genetic, epidemiologic, and pathophysiologic investigations; efforts to define genetic and nongenetic forms; expansion of the RLS Foundation collection at the Harvard Brain Tissue Resource Center; and studies of PLM as it relates to RLS.

THE CHALLENGE: WHAT WE NEED TO DISCOVER

Research scientists who want to help vanquish RLS can review research priorities in a guide provided by the RLS Foundation. The following are areas in need of further research.

EPIDEMIOLOGY

How many people suffer from RLS? How many are seriously affected? Are there significant variations by race, gender, or geographic location? What are the ages of onset? What is the percentage of genetically transmitted RLS versus other causes? What is the degree of association with nongenetic causes such as end-stage renal disease, lumbosacral disease, pregnancy, Parkinson's disease, and attention-deficit/hyperactivity disorder?

A lot of work lies ahead.

A study published in *Archives of Internal Medicine* concluded that "the prevalence of restless legs in the adult population is high. Restless legs may be associated with decreased well-being, emphasizing the need for further research and greater medical recognition of this condition."[10] In some areas, RLS may affect more than 10 percent of the adult population, making it one of the most common neurological disorders and even more common than such important chronic diseases as diabetes.

GENETICS

To what extent is RLS a familial disease? If you have it, what are the odds that your relatives also have it or will get it?

Efforts are under way to identify and study families with multiple affected individuals and to perform segregation analyses, to determine the mode of transmission of the hereditary form or forms of RLS. It is now clear that, at least for patients who have early-onset RLS, the disease runs in the family. Roughly two-thirds of such patients will have an affected first-degree family member. Segregation analysis, which examines how a disease might be inherited, has shown that there is likely to be a dominant gene to explain some familial RLS. (A dominant gene is one that is active even if a person receives only a single copy from one parent.) Researchers are closing in on such genes: already three locations on different chromosomes have been found that seem highly likely to harbor a gene affecting RLS.[11]

NEUROPHYSIOLOGY

Which area, or areas, of the nervous system are affected in RLS? And what are the neurophysiologic correlates in individuals with RLS and PLM? Those with RLS and not PLM? Those with PLM and not RLS?

IRON

To what extent, and under what circumstances, does iron (or ferritin) play a role in RLS? Studies exist, but much more remains to be learned about the correlation between RLS and the storage of iron and its transport within the central nervous system.

Research in this area was advanced by the aforementioned formation of the RLS Foundation collection at the Harvard Brain Tissue Resource Center. As we saw in Chapter 5, an early study employing tissue from the collection confirmed an altered state of iron storage in the critical motor area of the brain.

CIRCADIAN RHYTHMS

Why do RLS and PLM strike at night, depriving victims of treasured sleep? The reason is that the symptoms of some diseases, like asthma, are triggered by the workings of an internal clock. This clock produces *circadian rhythms,* changes in the levels of a substance or activity of a biological process that vary over the course of a day and night and then repeat that variation similarly day after day. That's the same process that causes the leaves of certain plants to close at night and that cause your pulse rate, blood pressure, and body temperature to fall at night. Basic as they are, there is still much to be learned about circadian rhythms, especially as related to RLS.

The RLS Foundation encourages scientists "to identify, quantify, and correlate the role of circadian rhythms in RLS by measuring biologic markers associated with circadian rhythms and correlating these measures with symptom severity and treatment effects."

DOPAMINE

We need to learn more about the role of this crucial neurotransmitter. Since we know that dopamine is critically involved in both RLS and Parkinson's disease, it would be beneficial for neurologists who study Parkinson's to also study RLS and PLM. What is learned from Parkinson's disease may offer clues to the causation of RLS, and vice versa. Speaking about a similar cross-benefit, an NIH document opined: "Parkinson's disease research can lead the way in the fight against all forms of neurodegeneration. The converse is also true. Research on other types of neurodegeneration may provide vital clues to curing Parkinson's disease." While RLS is definitely not a neurodegenerative disorder, the same principle of mutual discovery holds between Parkinson's disease and RLS.

TREATMENT MODEL

The treatment of RLS will be improved to the degree to which the effects of certain drugs are evaluated, whether in test tubes or by using an animal model, or with advanced imaging technology.

AN ADHD CONNECTION?

An increasing number of researchers are convinced that there is a connection between RLS or PLM and attention-deficit/hyperactivity disorder. (ADHD is a genetic, biochemical disorder characterized by inattention, restlessness, distractibility, and impulsivity.) This belief, if verified, would have far-reaching implications in the study of brain disorders, especially if it turns out that both disorders are caused by reduced activity of the dopaminergic system and respond well to drugs that promote dopamine action.

According to one study, "A patient with ADHD or his or her family may be more likely to also have RLS."[12]

I first heard about the possibility of an ADHD/RLS link from Dr. Joseph Lipinski Jr., of the Medical University of South Carolina, who along with Drs. Walters and Picchietti did pioneering work in the field. Until recently RLS and ADHD research concentrated on children, but a study presented at the 2001 American Academy of Neurology annual meeting showed that adults with RLS are more likely to have ADHD than are adults who don't have the disorder.[13]

Research on RLS and ADHD is limited because neither affliction can be measured by instruments. Nonetheless, evidence gathered in the more numerous studies of children does seem to establish comorbidity of RLS or PLM and ADHD. Dr. Picchietti said at the meeting that he and his colleagues "were amazed to discover that many kids who had been referred for ADHD turned out to have sleep problems," and that 25 to 50 percent of them had PLM, which *can* be measured with polysomnographic instruments.[14]

Writings about this intriguing possibility are tentative and call for more research. A study in 1998 concluded that "at the very least PLM might simply be associated with ADHD or, alternatively, that PLM and RLS can contribute to the inattentiveness and hyperactivity in a subgroup of children diagnosed as having ADHD. However, this study showed only co-occurrence of these sleep disorders with ADHD. Further work will be necessary to determine if they truly can cause or aggravate ADHD symptomatology."[15] Dr. William Ondo believes "a subset of ADHD *is* RLS, so they are clearly related. I think RLS is misdiagnosed as ADHD sometimes in kids because RLS certainly occurs in kids and may mimic ADHD symptoms. They want to get up and walk around."

In a study published in December 2005 in *Annals of Neurology*, Mayo Clinic researchers concluded that, for thirty-two patients with childhood-onset RLS, twenty-four (72 percent) had serum ferritin levels below 50 mg/L and twenty-three had a strong family connection to RLS. Suresh Kotagal, MD, professor of neurology at Mayo Clinic College of Medicine, Rochester, Minnesota, said he has noticed that about a third of the children he sees for ADHD, which accounts for the childhood onset, also have underlying RLS symptoms. "There are also some short but important case reports of children with ADHD and RLS that [show that] as you treat RLS, the daytime symptoms of inattentiveness, hyperactivity, and oppositional behavior seem to settle down."[16]

A LOT TO LEARN ABOUT GENES

No area of RLS investigation holds more promise, or presents greater difficulties, than genetics. Years of research have finally presented scientists with a genetic map, the genome, but the task of discerning the road to a cure for familial RLS remains arduous.

Recent research indicates that nearly 50 percent of RLS cases may be genetic. Early studies by RLSF Scientific Advisory Board member Dr. Jacques Montplaisir, of the Hospital of the Sacred Heart in Montreal, and his colleague Dr. R. Godbout gave the impression that these cases were the most severe, but further studies by the same researchers failed to confirm that idea. These later studies did, however, seem to demonstrate an earlier age of onset for familial RLS.[17]

Until recently, a lack of funds hampered researchers looking into the genetic role in RLS, but research financing has improved somewhat thanks to the RLS Foundation, its distinguished Scientific Advisory Board, the National Institutes of Health, and the scientific and medical community's increased interest in the disease. This interest is also reflected in the increasing number of articles on genetic studies in medical journals.

Gerald D. Fischbach, MD, former director of the National Institute of Neurological Disorders and Stroke, sees the possibility of genetics leading to a cure. At the November 11, 1999, Dopamine Connection Workshop, Dr. Fischbach said:

> One of the most important priorities in RLS research is to identify a gene or genes that may cause or act as a risk factor for RLS. Once we find the genetic abnormality behind RLS, we can focus on reproducing the disorder in animals. That will enable us to study proteins that are involved and to come up with a way to correct the abnormality.

Understanding familial forms of these diseases will take time. Indeed, there is a long way to go in the search for a genetic culprit, but for the first time, at the beginning of the twenty-first century, important genetic studies are in progress.

How to sum up where we now stand? Let's paraphrase Winston Churchill: "This is not the end. It may not even be the beginning of the end. But it is, probably, the end of the beginning."

When a cure is found, and RLS is but a hard-to-describe memory, it is to be hoped that great credit will be given to those who worked so hard to help the afflicted. Credit on that victorious day should of course go to the medical community, but also to those volunteers who gave time, energy, money, and imagination to the quest. If all who deserve inclusion were in this book, it would be impossibly long. They all have my admiration and gratitude.

NOTES

Introduction

1. Robert Yoakum, "Night Walkers: Restless Legs Syndrome," *Modern Maturity* (September-October 1994): 54.
2. C. Earley, "Restless Legs Syndrome," *New England Journal of Medicine* 348 (May 2003): 2103–9.
3. Janet Farrar Worthington, "Rest for the Weary," *Hopkins Medical News* (Fall 1991).
4. Drugs that can worsen RLS include

   antidepressants, such as Elavil, Prozac, Paxil
   antihistamines: cold and allergy preparations
   antiemetics, such as Compazine, Reglan
   lithium, such as Eskalith, Lithobid, Lithonate, Lithotabs
   calcium channel blockers (prescribed for heart disease and hypertension)
   major tranquilizers, such as Haldol and phenothiazines (Trilafon,
     Thorazine, etc.)

   From *Restless Legs Syndrome (RLS) and Periodic Limb Movement Disorder (PLMD)*, a wellness booklet (Westchester, IL: American Academy of Sleep Medicine, 2000).

Chapter 1: Yes, It Is a Real Disease

1. In *Complete Essays of Montaigne* (Palo Alto, CA: Stanford University Press, 1958).

2. Thomas Willis, *The London Practice of Physick* (London: Bassett, Dring, Harper, and Crook, 1683). Available at www.allbookstores.com/book/ 0893415057.

3. Worldwide Education and Awareness for Movement Disorders, www .wemove.org/glossary.

4. Karl A. Ekbom, "Restless Legs: A Clinical Study," *Acta Medica Scandinavica* 158 (1945): 1–123.

5. A. Desautels, G. Turecki, J. Montplaisir, A. Sequira, A. Verner, and G. A. Rouleau, "Identification of a Major Susceptibility Locus for Restless Legs Syndrome on Chromosome 12q," *American Journal of Human Genetics* 69 (2001): 1266–70.

6. J. W. Winkelman, "Restless Legs Syndrome in ESRD," *Nephrology News & Issues* 11 (Nov. 13, 1999): 27, 31, 32.

7. D. Nichols, R. Allen, J. Grauke, J. Brown, M. Rice, P. Hyde, W. Dement, and C. Kushida, "Restless Legs Syndrome Symptoms in Primary Care: A Prevalence Study," *Archives of Internal Medicine* 163 (2003): 2323.

8. Ibid., 2323–29.

9. Ibid.

10. E. Johnson, *Omnibus Sleep in America Poll* (Washington, DC: National Sleep Foundation, 2005).

11. E. Johnson, *Omnibus Sleep in America Poll* (Washington, DC: National Sleep Foundation, 1999, 2000, 2001, 2002, 2003).

12. "Largest-Ever Multinational Study Confirms that RLS Is Profoundly Underdiagnosed and a Deeply Disruptive Sleep Disorder," *NightWalkers* Summer 2004, 2.

Chapter 2: Eighteen Years: The Misdiagnosis of RLS

1. "Restless Legs: It's No Laughing Matter," *NightWalkers* (February 2001): 13.

2. Johnson, *Omnibus Sleep in America Poll*, 2003.

3. William C. Dement, Health & Environment Subcommittee Hearing, *New Developments in Medical Research: NIH & Patient Groups; Public Policy Recommendations to the U.S. Congress from the National Commission on Sleep Disorders Research (1990–1992), 1998 Update* (Mar. 26, 1998): 6. See www .stanford.edu/~dement/testimony.html.

4. Ibid., 4.

5. Ibid., 12.

6. Ibid., 6.

7. Ibid.

8. Ibid., 3.

9. *Sleep in America: 2005*, National Sleep Foundation–Gallup Poll (March 2005): 35.

10. Dement, Health & Environment Subcommittee Hearing, *New Developments in Medical Research.*

Chapter 3: Do I Have RLS?

1. A. Walters, "The International Restless Legs Syndrome Study Group: Toward a Better Definition of the Restless Legs Syndrome," *Movement Disorders* 10 (1995): 634–42; R. Allen, D. Picchietti, W. Hening, C. Trenkwalder, A. Walters, and J. Montplaisir, "Restless Legs Syndrome: Diagnostic Criteria, Special Considerations, and Epidemiology: A Report from the Restless Legs Syndrome Diagnosis and Epidemiology Workshop at the National Institutes of Health," *Sleep Medicine* 4 (2003): 101–19.

2. C. P. Symonds, "Nocturnal myoclonus," *Journal of Neurology, Neurosurgery, and Psychiatry* 16 (1953): 166–71; E. Lugaresi, C. A. Tassinari, G. Coccagna, and C. Ambrosetto, "Particularités cliniques et polygraphiques du syndrome d'impatience des membres inférieurs," *Revue Neurologique* 113 (1965): 545–55.

3. William Attwood, *Making It Through Middle Age* (New York: Atheneum, 1982).

4. K. Berger, J. Luedemann, C. Trenkwalder, U. John, and C. Kessler, "Sex and the Risk of Restless Legs Syndrome in the General Population," *Archives of Internal Medicine* 164 (2004): 196–202.

5. Nichols et al., "Restless Legs Syndrome Symptoms in Primary Care," 2326.

Chapter 4: Sleep and How to Get More of It

1. National Institute of Neurological Disorders and Stroke, *Brain Basics: Understanding Sleep* (Bethesda, MD: NIH Publication No. 04-3440, October 2004).

2. *Sleep in America: 2005*, National Sleep Foundation–Gallup Poll (March 2005): 35.

3. Arlene Weintraub, "I Can't Sleep," *BusinessWeek*, January 26, 2004, 69.

4. William C. Dement and Christopher Vaughan, *The Promise of Sleep* (New York: Delacorte Press, 1999): 5.

5. U.S. Surgeon General Richard H. Carmona, "Opening Remarks: Frontiers of Knowledge in Sleep and Sleep Disorders: Opportunities for Improving Health and Quality of Life," National Institutes of Health, Bethesda, MD, Mar. 29, 2004, 1.

6. Johnson, *Omnibus Sleep in America Poll*, 2005: 18.

7. Ibid., 7.

8. "Sleep Debt and Its Ravages," *BusinessWeek*, Jan. 26, 2004, 69.

9. Kelly Greene, "Aging Well: Growing Older Doesn't Have to Mean Sleeping Less," *Wall Street Journal*, November 11, 2002, R10.

10. Dement and Vaughan, *The Promise of Sleep*, 260.

11. National Commission on Sleep Disorders Research, *Wake Up America: A National Sleep Alert* (Washington, DC: Government Printing Office, 1993).

12. Dement and Vaughan, *The Promise of Sleep*, 261–62.

13. "Sleep Debt and Its Ravages."

14. Johnson, *Omnibus Sleep in America Poll*, 2005.

15. Dement and Vaughan, *The Promise of Sleep*, 123. William C. Dement, a world-renowned sleep expert, is also known, although in a far more limited circle, as a jazz musician. His enthusiasm for jazz led him to the following observation about the rhythm of successful sleep:

> When one player just can't swing with the rest of the group, it makes the whole thing hard for everyone. Everything seems effortless when the whole band is jamming, but one out-of-rhythm musician . . . just makes it hard, exhausting

work. In the same way, when people are out of rhythm with their sleep cycles, or when a large sleep debt is dragging them down, it makes everything in life so hard.

When sleep works—and when we allow it to work—our minds and bodies are in tune and working together. . . . Sleep bolsters us in countless ways, augmenting our feelings of happiness and vitality [permitting us] to reach our potential for creativity, productivity, and learning. (p. 73)

16. Johnson, *Omnibus Sleep in America Poll,* 2005, 5.
17. *The search for sleep is as old as humankind.* In 1894, the editor of the *British Medical Journal* quoted a number of techniques from the *Glasgow Herald:*

"Soap your head with the ordinary yellow soap; rub it into the roots of the hair until your head is just lather all over, tie it up in a napkin, go to bed, and wash it out in the morning. Do this for a fortnight. Take no tea after 6 p.m. I did this, and have never been troubled with sleeplessness since. I have lost sleep on an occasion since, but one or two nights of the soap cure put it all right. I have conversed with medical men, but I have had no explanation from any of them. All that I am careful about is that it cured me."

We cannot help thinking that some of our sleepless readers would prefer the disease to the cure. But if any should like to try it, may we advise that they should first, at any rate, follow that part of the advice which relates to the tea, and leave the soap part as a last resource.

Chapter 5: Medical Help

1. Sandra Blakeslee, "How Brain May Weigh the World with Simple Dopamine System," *New York Times,* Mar. 19, 1996.
2. At the November 10–11, 1999, Dopamine Connection workshop, Dr. Hyman called attention to a neglected aspect of dopamine function: its long-term effects.

He pointed out that dopamine, when transmitting information from neuron to neuron by binding to its receptors, simultaneously exerts two kinds of actions.

First, it initiates rapid changes in the cells' membranes. This leads to a change in their responses to other neurotransmitters. Second, dopamine initiates complex biochemical changes within those cells—changes that ultimately alter their biochemical properties.

Because dopamine involves such widely distributed actions across the brain, it's understandable that a variety of symptoms are seen when it malfunctions. With respect to restless legs syndrome specifically, the possibility of long-term cellular changes raises questions about the origins of the syndrome—and possible side effects from the regular use of dopaminergic medications. Perhaps the best illustration of the long-term actions of dopamine comes from research on the way normal memory is formed. Diverse approaches clearly demonstrate that dopamine is required for the formation of multiple forms of long-term memory.

Proper formation of spatial memories also requires dopamine, acting in a brain structure called the hippocampus. What sometimes have been called habit memories are laid down in another brain region, the striatum—again involving the actions of dopamine.

Finally, dopamine plays a crucial role in creating the shorter-term form of memory called working memory, which takes place in the prefrontal cerebral cortex.

Other evidence that dopamine produces long-term effects on brain function comes from the study of people with Parkinson's disease who are on long-term L-dopa therapy. In the absence of normal dopamine-producing cells, neurons in the striatum become supersensitive to the effects of dopamine.

Exposure to intermittent dopamine stimulation can lead to a range of behavioral symptoms, including abnormal involuntary movements and psychotic symptoms, along with such side effects as nausea, hypotension, rhinitis, and hallucinations. All of these clearly limit the utility of dopamine therapy.

The ultimate goal of this research is to understand ways in which abnormal dopamine patterns contribute to RLS and other disorders. Researchers can then design therapies that target the apparent dopamine-related irregularities that play a role in RLS.

"With an ability to target medications to act in restricted brain regions," Dr. Hyman concluded, "we will expect to avoid the adverse side effects that make current treatment unsuitable for a substantial number of patients with RLS."

3. Karl Ekbom, "Restless Legs Syndrome," *Neurology* 10 (1960): 872.

4. A. Walters, J. Winkelman, C. Trenkwalder, J. M. Fry, V. Kataria, M. Wagner, R. Sharma, and W. Hening, "Long-Term Follow-up on Restless Legs Syndrome Patients Treated with Opioids," *Movement Disorders* 16 (2001): 1105–9.

5. Ibid.

6. Charles Cleeland, "Undertreatment of Cancer Pain in Elderly Patients," *Journal of American Medical Association* 279 (1998): 1914–15.

7. Walters et al., "Long-Term Follow-up."

8. Diego Garcia-Borreguero, O. Larrosa, Y. de la Llave, K. Verger, X. Masramon, and G. Hernandez, "Treatment of Restless Legs Syndrome with Gabapentin: A Double-Blind Crossover Study," *Neurology* 59 (2002): 1573–79.

9. M. H. Silber, B. L. Ehrenberg, R. P. Allen, M. J. Buchfuhrer, C. J. Earley, W. A. Hening, and D. B. Rye, "An Algorithm for the Management of Restless Legs Syndrome," *Mayo Clinic Proceedings* 79 (2004): 916–22.

10. K. Stiasny, J. Robbecke, P. Schuler, and W. H. Oertel, "Treatment of Idiopathic Restless Legs Syndrome (RLS) with the D2-agonist Cabergoline: An Open Clinical Trial," *Sleep* 23 (2000): 349–54.

11. N. Nordlander, "Therapie in Restless Legs," *Acta Neurologica Scandinavica* 145 (1953): 453–57. Ekbom, "Restless Legs Syndrome," 868–73.

12. Winkelman, "Restless Legs Syndrome in ESRD," *Nephrology News & Issues* 1999.

13. Annual Data System Report, US Renal Data System, 2002. Available at www.usrds.org/adr.htm.

14. J. W. Winkelman, G. M. Chertow, and J. M. Lazarus, "Restless Legs Syndrome in End-Stage Renal Disease," *American Journal of Kidney Diseases* 28 (1996): 372–78.

15. K. Ekbom, "Restless Legs: A Clinical Study."

16. The article has been lightly edited for inclusion here. Bruce Ehrenberg, "Pregnancy and RLS/PLMS," *NightWalkers,* August 1997.

Chapter 7: Coping

1. A. H. Kanter, "The Effect of Sclerotherapy on Restless Legs Syndrome," *Dermatologic Surgery* 21 (1995): 328–32.
2. Johnson, *Omnibus Sleep in America Poll,* 2005.
3. Pickett Guthrie, "Does the Sleep Thief Have a Special Grudge against Women?" presented at RLS Foundation National Meeting, Long Beach, CA, Nov. 14, 2004.

Chapter 8: Special Challenges

1. "Chronic Stress Can Cripple, Cause Illness, Experts Say," *Waterbury Republican,* Oct. 30, 1997.
2. S. Sevim, O. Dogu, M. Aral, O. Metin, and H. Camdeverin, "Correlation of Anxiety and Depression Symptoms in Patients with Restless Legs Syndrome: A Population-Based Survey," *Journal of Neurology, Neurosurgery, & Psychiatry* 75 (2004): 226–30.
3. National Center on Sleep Disorders Research, National Heart, Lung, and Blood Institute, National Institutes of Health, *Restless Legs Syndrome: Detection and Management in Primary Care* (Bethesda, MD: NIH Publication No. 00-3788, March 2000).
4. Weintraub, "I Can't Sleep," 69.
5. "Commission Report Puts Sleep Research in the Spotlight," *Somniloquy* 6 (1994): 3.
6. "Don't Doze and Drive," *Harvard Health Letter* (October 1998): 8.
7. Sandy Rovner, "The Danger in Driving Drowsy," *Washington Post Health,* January 10, 1995, HV13.
8. Robert Pear, "U.S. Toughens Enforcement of Nursing Home Standards," *New York Times,* Dec. 4, 2000, A21.

Chapter 9: Hope

1. T. Wittmaack, *Pathologie und Therapie der Sensibilitat-Neurosen* (Leipzig: Schafer, 1861), 459.
2. R. Bing, *Lehrbuch der Nervenkrankheiten* (Berlin: 1913).
3. H. Oppenheim, *Lehrbuch der Nervenkrankheiten,* 7th ed. (Berlin: S. Karger, 1923).

4. J. D. Mussio-Fournier and F. Rawak, "Familiares Auftreten von Pruritis, Urtikaria und Parasthetischer Hyperkinese der Unteren Extremitaten," *Confinia Neurological* 3 (Switzerland) (1940): 110–14.

5. F. G. Allison, "Obscure Pains in the Chest, Back or Limbs," *Canadian Medical Association Journal* 48 (1943): 36.

6. S. Ancoli-Israel, A. R. Seifert, and M. Lemon, "Thermal Biofeedback and Periodic Movements in Sleep: Patients' Subjective Report and a Case Study," *Biofeedback and Self-Regulation* 86 (1986): 177.

7. C. P. Symonds, "Nocturnal Myoclonus," *Journal of Neurology, Neurosurgery, & Psychiatry* 16 (1953): 166; E. Lugaresi, G. Coccagna, D. Gambi, et al., "A Propos de Quelques Manifestations Nocturnes Myocloniques (Nocturnal Myoclonus de Symonds), *Revista de Neurología* 115 (Spain) (1966): 547; E. Lugaresi, C. A. Tassinari, G. Coccagna, et al., "Particularités Cliniques et Polygraphiques du Syndrome d'Impatience des Membres Inférieurs," *Revista de Neurología* 113 (1965): 545.

8. An intriguing example of research done at the University of Bologna was published by Giorgio Coccagna and Elio Lugaresi as "The Friar's Tale," in Virginia Wilson, *Sleep Thief: Restless Legs Syndrome* (Orange Park, FL: Galaxy Books, 1996).

9. A. S. Walters, "Toward a Better Definition of the Restless Legs Syndrome: The International Restless Legs Syndrome Study Group," *Movement Disorders* 10 (1995): 634–42.

10. B. Phillips, T. Young, L. Finn, K. Asher, W. A. Hening, and C. Purvis, "Epidemiology of Restless Legs Syndrome in Adults," *Archives of Internal Medicine* 160 (2000): 2137.

11. For insight into how researchers are pursuing a genetic key to RLS, see the abstract of Christopher Earley's grant from the National Institute of Aging, "Determining the Genetics of RLS," at www.neuro.jhmi.edu/rls/research.htm.

12. M. Wagner, A. Walters, and B. Fisher, "Symptoms of Attention-Deficit/Hyperactivity Disorder in Adults with Restless Legs Syndrome," *Sleep* 27 (2004): 1499–1504.

13. Ibid.

14. Picchietti became aware of RLS in the early 1980s, when few doctors had even heard of the disease. In an interview circa 2000 with the author, he told

how he diagnosed his wife after coming across the syndrome in a book on rare neurological diseases. "She had gone to a doctor with the problem as an adolescent but had been told she had growing pains. The plot thickened when I discovered in the course of a sleep test in 1984 that her father had severe RLS."

A few years later Dr. Arthur Walters signed the family up for a study trying to track down a gene for RLS. "Beginning with our children—all three had RLS—we could trace the gene back five generations."

I asked Picchietti about the emotional consequences for a family of having both parents and children afflicted. "It puts some unique stresses on families when you have children who don't sleep well," he replied. "Kids need more sleep than adults. When they don't get it, the result can be a pretty vicious cycle of sleep deprivation. That's particularly true if, as is likely, one of the parents has RLS. The odds are that the afflicted parent would also have PLMD, keeping the other parent awake if they sleep in the same bed."

15. D. L. Picchietti, S. J. England, A. S. Walters, K. Willis, and T. Verrico, "Periodic Limb Movement Disorder and Restless Legs Syndrome in Children with Attention-Deficit Hyperactivity Disorder," *Journal of Child Neurology* 13 (1998): 593.

16. S. Kotagal and M. H. Silber, "Childhood-Onset Restless Legs Syndrome," *Annals of Neurology* 56 (2004): 803–7.

17. J. Winkelman, T. C. Wetter, S. Collado, T. Gasser, M. Dichgans, A. Yassouridis, et al., "Clinical Characteristics and Frequency of the Hereditary Restless Legs Syndrome in a Population of 300 Patients," *Sleep* 23 (2000): 597–602.

RLS MILESTONES

1672	First recorded description of RLS by English physician Sir Thomas Willis.
1913	R. Bing described a form of bone paresthesia and identified it as anxietas tibiarum.
1923	H. Oppenheim was apparently the first to define RLS as a neurologic disorder.
1941	J. D. Mussio-Fournier and F. Rawak described the clinical features of RLS. They correctly believed it was a disorder of the central nervous system. They also concluded that the ailment could be transmitted genetically and that it appeared with unexpected frequency during pregnancy.
1943	F. G. Allison, a Canadian physician who suffered from RLS himself, wrote the first description of the associated syndrome now known as periodic limb movement (PLM).
1945	First comprehensive and systematic clinical description of RLS, by Swedish neurologist Karl A. Ekbom, who described many clinical aspects—including familial features, epidemiology, and therapy—and named the disorder restless legs syndrome.
1947–53	French researchers M. Bonduelle and B. Jolivet concluded (as did

Ekbom at about the same time) that RLS was often caused by circulatory disruptions.

1953   Description of nocturnal myoclonus by C. P. Symonds.

1966   Dr. Elio Lugaresi and Italian colleagues were the first to record periodic leg movements during polysomnographic studies and associated this phenomenon (PLMD, which they called nocturnal myoclonus) with RLS.

1976   Emphasis of waking involuntary movements and family association by D. Boghen and J. Peyronnard.

1976–82   Careful clinical and epidemiologic studies of PLMD by the Weissman group, especially N. Coleman and Christian Guilleminault.

1978–82   Initial descriptions of Klonopin (clonazepam) as effective in RLS and PLMD.

1980s   Initial modern descriptions of effectiveness of opioids and dopaminergic agents in RLS and PLMD by S. Akpinar, Jacques Montplaisir, and Arthur Walters.

1992   Establishment of RLS Foundation.

1993   Medical Advisory Board established by the RLS Foundation.

1993–97   Evaluation of effectiveness and drawbacks of levodopa and dopamine agonists led by Richard Allen, P. M. Becker, Claudia Trenkwalder, and Jacques Montplaisir groups.

1994   International RLS Study Group founded by Arthur Walters, resulting in first international conference on RLS.

1994   First RLS Foundation support group established, in Seattle, Washington, by Juanita Therrell.

1994   Participation of RLS Foundation in educational efforts of the Associated Professional Sleep Societies and the American Academy of Neurology, led by Richard Allen and Wayne Hening.

1995   Initial paper of RLS International Study group proposing standard definition of RLS.

1995   First report of usefulness of antiseizure medicine Neurontin (gabapentin) in RLS.

1995–97   Series of epidemiologic and family studies, both showing high prevalence and confirming strong familial association of RLS.

1997   Conference held at the National Academy of Sciences. Establish-
         ment of RLS Foundation Scientific Advisory Board.

1998   House and Senate Appropriations Subcommittees, which fund the
         Department of Health and Human Services (parent of National In-
         stitutes of Health), included the following language in their reports:

> Restless legs syndrome. The Committee encourages NINDS (National
> Institute for Neurological Disorder and Stroke) to follow up on recent
> scientific publications highlighting the public health significance of
> Restless Legs Syndrome (RLS) and Periodic Limb Movement Disor-
> der (PLMD). Any research conducted should include studies which
> investigate the relation of RLS and PLMD to other conditions such as
> pregnancy, diabetes, renal disease, fibromyalgia, spinal cord injuries,
> neuropathies, and attention-deficit/hyperactivity disorder and should
> be coordinated with the appropriate Institutes.

1999   Major scientific figures participate in NIH workshop entitled The
         Dopamine Connection in Restless Legs Syndrome, Periodic Limb
         Movement Disorder, Parkinsonism, and Narcolepsy: Toward a Bet-
         ter Understanding of Common Mechanisms in Uncommon Disor-
         ders.

1999   First standards for management of RLS, by American Academy of
         Sleep Medicine.

2000   RLS Foundation collection established at the Harvard Brain Tissue
         Resource Center.

2001   Program announcement (PA) from the NIH for research on RLS.

2001   First genetic linkage in RLS identified by RLS Foundation–funded
         researchers.

2004   Expansion of RLS Foundation research programs funded by the
         National Institute for Neurological Disorder and Stroke.

2005   GlaxoSmithKline markets the first medication approved for RLS/
         PLMD use.

GLOSSARY

ADHD (Attention-Deficit/Hyperactivity Disorder) A genetic, biochemical disorder characterized by inattention, restlessness, distractibility, and impulsivity.

agonist A drug that binds to a receptor of a cell and triggers a response by the cell. An agonist often mimics the action of a naturally occurring substance. An agonist produces an action. It is the opposite of an antagonist, which acts against and blocks an action. Agonists and antagonists are key agents in the chemistry of the human body.

akathisia A neurologic condition of motor restlessness, manifested by a sensation of muscular quivering, an urge to constantly move about, and an inability to sit still.

akinesia Absence of movement or loss of the ability to move, as in temporary or prolonged paralysis or "freezing in place."

anemia Too few red blood cells in the bloodstream, resulting in insufficient oxygen to tissues and organs.

antagonist Drug that binds to a cell receptor or a hormone, a neurotransmitter, or another drug, and thus blocks the action of the other substance without producing any physiological effect itself.

augmentation Sometimes referred to as "toleration." When applied to RLS, it involves a progressively earlier daily onset of symptoms. The symptoms may be more intense and may also be experienced beyond the legs—in the trunk or arms. May occur as a result of the use of certain medications (particularly levodopa), especially among those who have severe symptoms or are taking high doses of the drug.

autosomal dominant disorder Human traits, such as an individual's eye color, hair color, or expression of certain diseases, result from the interaction of one gene inherited from the father and one gene from the mother. In autosomal dominant disorders, the presence of a single copy of a mutated gene may result in the disease. In other words, the mutated gene may dominate or "override" the instructions of the normal gene on the other chromosome, potentially leading to disease expression. Individuals with an autosomal dominant disease trait have a 50 percent risk of transmitting the mutated gene to their children.

autosomal recessive disorder With autosomal recessive disorders, two copies of the disease gene must be inherited in order for an individual to potentially develop the disease. If both the mother and father carry a copy of the disease gene, each child has a 25 percent risk of inheriting the two genes for the disease. There is a 50 percent risk that the children may inherit one copy of the disease gene and be carriers for the disease trait (heterozygous carriers). In addition, there is a 25 percent chance that the parents' offspring will inherit two normal copies of the gene and will neither develop the disorder nor be carriers for this disease trait.

axons Nerve fibers. Axons are the relatively slender extensions of neurons that transmit nerve impulses away from nerve cell bodies. The ends of the axons or *terminals* release chemical substances known as neurotransmitters, enabling the transmission of nerve impulses to other neurons or effector organs. The whitish, fatty, protein-containing substance called *myelin* forms an insulating, protective, cylindrical sheath around some axons, serving to increase the speed and efficiency of nerve impulse transmissions.

basal ganglia Specialized nerve cell clusters of gray matter deep within each cerebral hemisphere and the upper brain stem, including the striate body (caudate and lentiform nuclei) and other cell groups such as the subthalamic nucleus and substantia nigra. The basal ganglia assist in initiating and regulating movement.

benzodiazepines A class of medications that act upon the central nervous system to reduce communication between certain neurons, lowering the level of activity in the brain. Benzodiazepines are effective in reducing anxiety, stress, or agitation; promoting sleep; alleviating restlessness; and relaxing muscles.

brain stem The region of the brain consisting of the medulla oblongata, pons, and midbrain. The brain stem primarily contains white matter interspersed with some gray matter. This area of the brain serves as a two-way conduction path, conveying nerve impulses between other brain regions and the spinal cord. In addition, most of the twelve pairs of cranial nerves from the brain arise from the brain stem, regulating breathing, digestion, heartbeat, blood pressure, pupil size, swallowing, and other basic functions.

cabergoline An ergotamine-based dopamine receptor agonist with a half-life of sixty-five hours. In the United States, it is marketed as Dostinex for the treatment of the rare disorder hyperprolactinemia, or high levels of the hormone prolactin.

carbidopa A drug that, when combined with levodopa, slows the peripheral breakdown of the levodopa, thereby allowing more of the levodopa to enter the brain.

carnitine A natural substance found in skeletal and cardiac muscle and the liver. Carnitine serves to transport fatty acids across mitochondrial membranes, thereby playing an important role in energy production and the metabolism of fatty acids.

cerebrospinal fluid (CSF) The fluid that flows through and protects the four cavities (ventricles) of the brain, the spinal cord's central canal, and the space (known as the subarachnoid space) between the middle and inner layers of the membrane (meninges) enclosing the brain and spinal cord. Laboratory analysis of CSF, usually obtained via lumbar puncture, may help to diagnose central nervous system infections, certain tumors, or particular neurological disorders. During lumbar puncture, CSF is removed from the spinal canal via a hollow needle inserted between certain bones of the spinal column within the lower back (usually the third and fourth lumbar vertebrae).

chromosome A structure in the nucleus containing a linear thread of DNA, which transmits genetic information.

circadian rhythm The regular recurrence, in cycles of about twenty-four hours, of biological processes or activities, such as sensitivity to drugs and stimuli, hormone secretion, sleeping, and feeding. This rhythm seems to be set by a "biological clock" that seems to be sensitive to alternating daylight and darkness.

clonus Movements characterized by alternate contractions and relaxations of a muscle, occurring in rapid succession. Clonus is frequently observed in conditions such as spasticity and certain seizure disorders.

corpus striatum The most important dopamine consumer for RLS (and Parkinson's) victims. In a central area of the brain, the striatum plays a major role in sending out commands for balance and coordination. Commands go from the nigral cells to the striatum cells, from the striatum cells to the spinal cord cells, from the spinal cord cells to the nerve networks, from the nerves to the muscles—all in an instant.

CSF transferrin Transferrin in the cerebrospinal fluid.

dopamine A substance in the body, a neurotransmitter that controls movement and balance and is essential to the proper functioning of the central nervous system (CNS). Dopamine assists in the effective transmission of electrochemical signals from one nerve cell (neuron) to another.

dopamine agonist (DA) A drug that acts like dopamine. DAs combine with dopamine receptors to mimic dopamine actions. Such medications stimulate dopamine receptors and produce dopamine-like effects.

dopamine autoreceptor A type of dopamine receptor that acts like a thermostat, preventing excess dopamine release as levels rise.

dopamine receptor A molecule on a receiving nerve cell (neuron) that is sensitive (or receptive) to stimulation (arousal) by dopamine or a dopamine agonist. At least five types have been identified, including D1, D2, D3 receptors and the dopamine autoreceptor.

dopamine receptor antagonist A pharmacologic agent that binds to and blocks the action of dopamine receptors, essentially hindering receptor activity by preventing stimulation by dopamine.

dopamine transporter A substance in the body that, after dopamine finishes sending its message, carries the dopamine back from the nerve ending to the cell that produced it so that the dopamine can be reused. The number of dopamine transporters is a sign of the number of nerve endings that produce or release dopamine.

dopaminergic Having the effect of dopamine or related to dopamine-producing cells.

dopaminergic dysfunction Malfunction of dopamine receptors.

dopaminergic uptake blocker An agent that blocks the uptake of dopamine at the synapse linking two cells.

double-blind trial A clinical experiment in which neither the patients nor the researchers are aware of which patients are receiving the active treatment and which are receiving a placebo.

dysarthria Disordered or impaired articulation of speech due to disturbances of muscular control, usually resulting from damage to the central or peripheral nervous system. Dysarthria is associated with certain neurodegenerative disorders, such as Parkinson's disease or Huntington's disease; cerebral palsy; brain tumors or stroke; or certain types of brain surgery.

dyskinesia The impairment of the power of voluntary movement, resulting in fragmentary or incomplete movements.

dyskinesias while awake (DWA) Uncontrolled, sporadic movements of the legs and, in some cases, the arms. These movements may be very rapid (myoclonic) or quite slow and prolonged (dystonic); they usually disappear upon voluntary action. Some researchers suspect that these movements may represent a wakeful form of periodic limb movements during sleep, or PLMS.

epidemiological study Examination of the distribution of disease as well as the determining factors related to specific diseases or health-related problems in a specific population.

epidemiology The study of the relationship of various factors determining the frequency and distribution of diseases in the human community.

ergot-derived medication A medication that has a chemical structure based on ergot, a plant alkaloid produced by a fungus called *Claviceps purpurea*. Permax and Parlodel are examples of ergot-derived medications that may be used to treat certain neurologic movement disorders.

estrogen (1) Any of several naturally occurring female sex hormones that promote the development of female secondary sexual characteristics and the proper functioning of the reproductive system; (2) synthetically produced agents used in birth control pills (oral contraceptives) or in the treatment of symptoms of menopause; osteoporosis, which is a bone disorder characterized by a progressive loss of bone mass; particular types of advanced post-menopausal breast cancer and prostate cancer; and other conditions.

ferritin A protein in the body that binds to iron; most of the iron stored in the body is attached to ferritin. Ferritin is found in the liver, spleen, skeletal muscles, and bone marrow. Only a small amount is found in the blood. The amount of ferritin in the blood indicates the amount of iron stored in the body.

Food and Drug Administration (FDA) Federal agency charged with ensuring that the food supply in the United States is safe and wholesome, that cosmetics are not harmful, and that medicines, medical devices, and radiation-emitting consumer products are safe and effective.

genes The smallest units of heredity. The information from all the genes, taken together, makes up the blueprint or plan for the human body and its functions. A gene is a short segment of DNA, which is interpreted by the body as a plan or template for building a specific protein.

half-life The time it takes for the blood level of a drug to decrease by half after a drug is stopped.

hereditary Inherited; inborn; referring to the genetic transmission of a trait, condition, or disorder from parent to offspring.

hippocampus A part of the limbic system also known as the "emotional brain" because it controls most of the involuntary aspects of emotional behavior related to survival: feelings of pleasure and pain such as anger, fear, and affection. The hippocampus is also involved in the processes of learning and memory.

idiopathic Of spontaneous origin; self-originated or of unknown cause. The term is derived from the prefix *idio-*, meaning one's own, and *pathos*, indicating disease.

myoclonus A neurologic movement disorder characterized by brief, involuntary, twitching, or shocklike contractions of a muscle or muscle group. These jerklike movements may be accompanied by periodic, unexpected interruptions in voluntary muscle contraction, leading to lapses of sustained posture (*negative myoclonus*). So-called positive and negative myoclonus are often seen in the same individuals and may affect the same muscle groups. Myoclonus is often a nonspecific finding, meaning that it may occur in the setting of additional neurologic abnormalities and be associated with any number of underlying conditions or disorders. In other patients, myoclonus appears as an isolated or a primary finding. Depending on the underlying cause and other factors, the shocklike muscle jerks may occur repeatedly or infrequently; may tend to appear under specific circumstances (e.g., with voluntary movements or in response to specific external sensory stimuli); and may affect any body region or regions.

nervous system The nervous system of the human body is divided into two interconnected systems: the central nervous system, which is made up of the brain and spinal cord, and the peripheral nervous system. The peripheral nervous system is further divided into the somatic nervous system (made up of peripheral nerve fibers that send sensory information to the central nervous system, and motor nerve fibers that project to skeletal muscle) and the autonomic nervous system.

neuroleptic An antipsychotic agent; the term refers to the effects on cognition and behavior of antipsychotic drugs, which produce a state of apathy, lack of initiative, and limited range of emotion and in psychotic patients cause a reduction in confusion and agitation and normalization of psychomotor activity.

neuron Any of the conducting cells of the nervous system. A typical neuron consists of a cell body, containing the nucleus and the surrounding cytoplasm; several short radiating connectors (dendrites); and one long connector (the axon), which terminates in twiglike branches (telodendrons) and may have branches (collaterals) projecting along its course.

neurotransmitter A specialized substance (such as norepinephrine or acetylcholine) that transfers nerve impulses across spaces between nerve cells (synapses). Neurotransmitters are naturally produced chemicals by which nerve cells communicate.

NIH The National Institutes of Health, among the world's foremost medical centers and a focal point for federal medical research. The NIH conduct research in their own laboratories, support the research of nonfederal scientists (like those working with the Restless Legs Syndrome Foundation, for example), help in the training of research investigators, and foster communication of medical information.

NREM sleep Non-REM (non–rapid eye movement) sleep, the normal period of dreamless, lighter sleep as compared to the deeper REM sleep. NREM sleep accounts for the major portion of sleep.

obstructive sleep apnea A sleep disorder characterized by episodes of temporary cessation of breathing due to obstruction of the airway.

opiate A drug derived from opium; a remedy containing or derived from opium; also any drug that induces sleep.

opioids Literally, "like or similar to opium"; refers to medications with opium-like effects, synthetic drugs that possess the characteristic properties of opiate narcotics but are not derived from opium.

paresthesias Abnormal sensations occurring spontaneously or in response to stimulation. Paresthesias may include prickling, tingling, burning, or tickling feelings; numbness; "pins and needles"; or cramplike sensations. Various neurologic movement disorders may be characterized by paresthesias, including restless legs syndrome (RLS), paroxysmal kinesigenic dyskinesia (PKD), and paroxysmal nonkinesigenic dyskinesia (PNKD).

Parkinson's disease (PD) A slowly progressive degenerative disorder of the central nervous system characterized by slowness or poverty of movement (bradykinesia), rigidity, postural instability, and tremor primarily while at rest. Additional characteristic findings include a shuffling, unbalanced manner of walking; forward bending or flexion of the trunk; a fixed or "masklike" facial expression; weakness of the voice; abnormally small, cramped handwriting (micrographia); and depression. Such abnormalities are thought to result from progressive loss of nerve cells within a certain region of the substantia nigra of the brain and the associated depletion of the neurotransmitter dopamine.

pathogenesis The origination and development of a disease.

periodic limb movement (PLM) A condition characterized by rhythmic movements of the limbs while awake or sleeping. The movements typically involve the legs, but upper extremity movements may also occur.

peripheral neuropathy Inflammation, degeneration, or damage of nerves of the peripheral nervous system (PNS). The PNS includes nerves that extend from the brain and spinal cord (central nervous system) to various parts of the body. Peripheral neuropathy may involve motor nerves, causing muscle weakness, and/or sensory nerves, resulting in pain, abnormal sensations such as numbness or tingling, or other findings.

polysomnography Simultaneous and continuous monitoring of relevant normal and abnormal physiological activity during sleep.

receptor A molecule on a neuron that receives a neurotransmitter. Reception of the neurotransmitter causes changes in the neuron that increase or decrease its likelihood of "firing," or sending its own signal to other neurons. Dopamine receptors are located on corpus striatum neurons and on nigral cells.

refractory Resistant to or not readily yielding to treatment.

REM sleep The period of sleep associated with dreaming, rapid eye movements (REM), and certain involuntary muscle movements.

restless legs syndrome (RLS) A neurologic movement disorder characterized by unusual, uncomfortable sensations (paresthesias/dysesthesias) deep within the calves and/or thighs, resulting in an irresistible urge to move the legs, and motor restlessness in response to or in an effort to alleviate discomfort. In some patients, the arms may also be affected. Symptoms become obvious or worse during periods of relaxation or inactivity; occur most frequently during the evening or the early part of the night; and may be temporarily relieved by voluntary movements of the affected area. Most patients experience associated sleep disturbances, including difficulties drifting off and remaining asleep. RLS is also often associated with periodic limb movements in sleep (PLMS). Episodes of PLMS typically occur during periods of NREM sleep.

restorative sleep A refreshing sleep, in which a person receives a sufficient amount of rest to feel refreshed and to engage in the activities of daily living without experiencing excessive daytime sleepiness (EDS).

RFA Request for applications.

sensorimotor Pertaining to both the sensory and motor aspects of a bodily function.

serotonin (3-[2-aminoethyl]-5-indolol) A vasoconstrictor found in many tissues of the body that is present in relatively high concentrations in portions of the central nervous system (e.g., hypothalamus, basal ganglia). Serotonin functions as a neurotransmitter, regulating the delivery of messages between nerve cells (neurons). This neurotransmitter is thought to play some role in regulating consciousness and mood states. Serotonin is also present in other tissues of the body such as the intestines and blood platelets.

serum ferritin Ferritin (a form of iron) in the blood.

sleep fragmentation A continual disruption of sleep, which often leads to excessive daytime sleepiness. This disruption can occur as the result of a variety of factors, including sleep disorders, the need to get up to use the bathroom, pain, and a noisy or uncomfortable sleeping environment.

sleep latency The interval of time between "settling in" to go to sleep and the onset of sleep.

sleep maintenance Once asleep, the ability to remain asleep.

SSRIs Selective serotonin reuptake inhibitors. Drugs belonging to this class are antidepressant agents that selectively inhibit the absorption of serotonin at certain nerve membranes (e.g., presynaptic neuronal membranes). These drugs increase the concentration of serotonin within the central nervous system and enhance serotonin's neurotransmission activities.

stimulus Something that creates a response in a muscle, nerve, gland, or other excitable tissue or organ of the body. The plural is *stimuli*.

substantia nigra A cell mass in the lower part of the brain, in which neurons manufacture dopamine.

synapse The junction between two neurons or between a neuron and an effector organ. As a nerve impulse reaches a synapse, the terminal or end of the *presynaptic* neuron's axon releases neurotransmitters, which diffuse across the gap and bind to receptors of the *postsynaptic* neuron or the effector organ (i.e., muscle or gland). As the electrical impulse is conducted across the gap, electrical changes are triggered that serve to continue or hinder transmission of the impulse.

Tourette's syndrome A neurologic disease of unknown cause that presents with multiple tics (uncontrolled behavior), associated with snorting, sniffing, and involuntary vocalizations.

uremia An excess of urea or other nitrogenous waste in the blood, most often due to renal failure.

Resources

The following organizations and websites provide additional information on restless legs syndrome.

American Academy of Sleep Medicine (AASM; formerly American Sleep Disorders Association)
One Westbrook Corporate Center, Suite 920
Westchester, IL 60154
www.aasmnet.org
tel: 708-492-0930

The AASM is a professional membership organization dedicated to the advancement of sleep medicine and related research. Its mission is to assure quality care for patients with sleep disorders, promote the advancement of sleep research, and provide public and professional education.

National Center on Sleep Disorders Research (NCSDR)
Two Rockledge Center, Suite 7024
6701 Rockledge Drive, MSC 7920
Bethesda, MD 20892-7920

tel: 301-435-0199

fax: 301-480-3451

The NCSDR supports research, scientist training, dissemination of health information, and other activities on sleep and sleep disorders.

National Heart, Lung, and Blood Institute (NHLBI) Information Center

PO Box 30105

Bethesda, MD 20824-0105

tel: 301-592-8573

fax: 240-629-3246

TTY (for people using adaptive equipment): 240-629-3255

The center acquires, analyzes, promotes, maintains, and disseminates programmatic and educational information related to sleep and sleep disorders. Write for a list of available publications.

National Sleep Foundation (NSF)

1522 K Street NW, Suite 500

Washington, DC 20005

nsf@sleepfoundation.org

www.sleepfoundation.org

fax: 202-347-3472

The NSF's goal is to increase public awareness about health problems related to sleep disorders. Information on programs such as the Drive Alert . . . Arrive Alive campaign and about the effects of sleep deprivation are on their web page.

Restless Legs Syndrome Foundation (RLSF)

819 Second Street SW

Rochester, MN 55902-2985

rlsfoundation@rls.org

www.rls.org

tel: 507-287-6465

fax: 507-287-6312

RLSF goals are to increase awareness of RLS, to improve treatments, and, through research, to find a cure. Their website lists support groups and provides brochures, newsletters, and other comprehensive information on RLS.

The National Institute of Neurological Disorders and Stroke (NINDS)
National Institutes of Health
Bethesda, MD 20892
www.ninds.nih.gov
tel: 800-352-9424 or 301-496-5751
TTY (for people using adaptive equipment): 301-468-5981

The mission of NINDS is to reduce the burden of neurological disease—a burden borne by every age group, by every segment of society, by people all over the world.

Support Groups

The numbers and websites below reflect information current at the time of publication. Since contact numbers and websites of groups and their leaders are subject to change, call the RLS Foundation at 507-287-6465 or go to www.rls.org.

• **Alabama**
Shoals Area Support Group
256-247-3171
NorthernAlabama@rlsgroups.org

• **Arizona**
Northwest Valley Support Group
623-566-2635
SunCity@rlsgroups.org

Payson RLS Support Group
928-468-6626
Payson@rlsgroups.org

Tucson NightWalkers
520-760-5039
Tucson@rlsgroups.org

• **Arkansas**
Arkansas RLS Support Group
501-223-9780
LittleRock@rlsgroups.org

Hot Springs Village Support Group
501-922-0049
HotSpringsVillage@rlsgroups.org

• **California**
Coachella Valley RLS Support Group
760-285-2231
CoachellaValley@rlsgroups.org

Gold Country Support Group
530-888-6026
Roseville@rlsgroups.org

Marin County RLS Support Group
415-456-0257
MarinCounty@rlsgroups.org

Monterey Bay Support Group
831-484-9058
MontereyBay@rlsgroups.org

North San Diego/La Jolla Support Group
760-489-1201
SanDiegoCounty@rlsgroups.org

RLS Support Group for Napa & Sonoma Counties
707-945-0779
Napa@rlsgroups.org

Shasta County CA RLS Support Group
916-336-5486
ShastaCounty@rlsgroups.org

South Sacramento County RLS Support Group
916-682-5209
Sacramento@rlsgroups.org

Sleep Starved of So. Orange County Support Group
949-551-5449
Soorangecounty@rlsgroups.org

Southern California Support Group
714-633-0123
SoCal@rlsgroups.org

• **Colorado**
Greater Denver Area Support Group
303-494-4913
Denver@rlsgroups.org

Northwest Colorado RLS Support Group
970-879-0284
NWColorado@rlsgroups.org

Southwest Colorado RLS Support Group
970-882-3888
SWColorado@rlsgroups.org

Western Colorado RLS Support Group
970-858-3520
WesternColorado@rlsgroups.org

• **Delaware**
Greater New Castle/Kent Support
302-292-2687
newcastlekent@rlsgroup.org

• **Florida**
Broward County Support Group
954-724-0438
BrowardCo@rlsgroups.org

Central Florida Support Group
352-259-0979
centralflorida@rlsgroups.org

Circadian Amblers
954-720-8034
Tamerac@rslgroups.org

Good Samaritan Village at
**   Kissimmee RLS Support Group**
None available
GoodSamaritanVillage@rlsgroups
    .org

North Florida/South Georgia RLS
**   Support Group**
904-573-8686
jacksonville@rlsgroups.org

North Tampa RLS Support Group
813-784-0603
NorthTampa@rlsgroups.org

South Florida Support Group
561-883-5956
BocaRaton@rlsgroups.org

Tampa Bay RLS Support Group
813-655-9000
TampaBay@rlsgroups.org

Treasure Coast RLS Support
**   Group**
772-546-0750
None available

• **Hawaii**
Honolulu Support Group
808-599-3788
Hawaii@rlsgroups.org

• **Illinois**
Central Illinois RLS Support
**   Group**
217-793-1703
Springfield@rslgroups.org

Champaign-Urbana RLS Support
**   Group**
217-586-3851
Champaign@rlsgroups.org

Heart of Illinois Support Group
Carol Mallard
309-353-2213
carolmallard@sbcglobal.net

Joliet RLS Support Group
815-372-1274
Joliet@rlsgroups.org

Southern Illinois RLS Support Group
618-942-7143
SouthernIllinois@rlsgroups.org

Southern Illinois RLS Support Group
618-568-1122
SouthernIllinois1@rlsgroups.org

• **Indiana**
Southern Indiana Support Group
812-522-2766
SouthernIndiana@rlsgroups.org

• **Iowa**
Central Iowa Support Group
515-597-2782
CentralIowa@rlsgroups.org

Central Iowa Support Group
515-388-4736
CentralIowa1@rlsgroups.org

Greater Omaha Support Group
712-566-2668
Omaha1@rlsgroups.org

• **Kansas**
South Central Kansas Support Group
316-773-5195
CentralKansas@rlsgroups.org

Kansas City RLS Support Group
913-268-8879
KansasCity@rlsgroups.org

• **Kentucky**
Central Kentucky Advocacy Education & Support Group
859-887-4109
Lexington@rlsgroups.org

Louisville Support Group
502-962-4653
Louisville@rlsgroups.org

Restless in Southern Kentucky
877-700-4070
Sokentucky@rlsgroups.org

• **Louisiana**
Capital Area Support Group
504-251-1950
BatonRouge@rlsgroups.org

• **Maine**
Central Maine Support Group
207-798-6787
Topsham@rlsgroups.org

Maine RLS Support Group
207-892-8391
SoMaine@rlsgroups.org

• **Maryland**
Baltimore Area Support Group
410-902-1818
Baltimore@rlsgroups.org

Baltimore Area Support Group
410-321-0349
Baltimore1@rlsgroups.org

• **Massachusetts**
South Shore Cape and Islands
   Support Group
508-790-7640
CapeCodW@rlsgroups.org

• **Michigan**
Mid Michigan RLS Support Group
817-980-4673
MidMichigan@rlsgroups.org

Western Michigan Support Group
616-532-1698
WesternMichigan@rlsgroups.org

• **Minnesota**
Northern MN RLS Support Group
218-328-5987
NorthernMinnesota@rlsgroups.org

Rochester Area Support Group
507-533-7864
SouthernMinnesota@rlsgroups.org

Twin Cities RLS Support Group
651-431-0349
StPaul@rslgroups.org

• **Mississippi**
Central Mississippi Support Group
601-267-0156
CentralMississippi@rslgroups.org

• **Missouri**
Central Missouri RLS Support
   Group
660-368-2382
CentralMissouri@rlsgroups.org

Mid Missouri Support Group
573-443-4436
MidMissouri@rlsgroups.org

• **Nebraska**
Greater Omaha Support Group
402-832-5177
Omaha@rlsgroup.org

Southeast Nebraska RLS Support
   Group
402-435-0172
Lincoln@rlsgroups.org

Southeast Nebraska Support Group
402-489-8075
Lincoln1@rlsgroups.org

• New Hampshire
Granite State RLS Support Group
603-225-2103
NewHampshire@rlsgroups.org

Greater Boston RLS Support
Group
603-926-9328
Seacoast@rlsgroups.org

Upper Valley NightWalkers
603-643-2624
UpperValley@rlsgroups.org

Upper Valley NightWalkers
603-448-3702
UpperValley1@rlsgroups.org

• New Jersey
Support Group of Central New
Jersey
908-756-1619
NewJersey@rlsgroups.org

• New York
Long Island RLS/PLMD Support
Group
631-225-0412
LongIsland@rlsgroups.org

Manhattan Support Group
212-233-0810
Manhattan@rlsgroups.org

Parkinson's Disease and Movement
Disorder Center
518-452-0914
Albany@rlsgroups.org

Western NY RLS Support Group
716-741-1560
Buffalo@rlsgroups.org

• North Carolina
Restless in Metrolina Support
Group
704-821-3832
Metrolina@rlsgroups.org

Restless in Raleigh Support Group
919-847-7506
Raleigh@rlsgroups.org

• Ohio
Central Ohio Support Group
None available
Columbus@rlsgroups.org

Maumee Valley RLS Support
Group
419-878-1716
MaumeeValley@rlsgroups.org

North East Ohio RLS Support Group
440-350-4567
Cleveland@rlsgroups.org

Southwestern Ohio Support Group
937-429-0620
SWOhio@rlsgroups.org

• Oregon
Portland Support Group
503-646-8925
Portland@rlsgroups.org

Southern Oregon RLS Support Group
541-955-2978
SouthernOregon@rlsgroups.org

• Pennsylvania
Bucks County RLS Group
215-504-0458
BucksCo@rlsgroups.org

Greater New Castle/Kent Support Group
215-641-4922
NewcastleKent1@rlsgroups.org

• Rhode Island
Southern Rhode Island RLS Support Group
401-322-3017
RhodeIsland@rlsgroups.org

• South Carolina
Greater Charleston / Low Country RLS Support Group
843-388-8006
CharlestonSC@comcast.net

Spartanburg Support Group
864-542-9706
Spartanburg@rlsgroups.org

• Tennessee
East Tennessee RLS Support Group
865-577-7215
Tennessee@rlsgroups.org

• Texas
Greater Dallas Support Group
972-422-0816
Dallas@rlsgroups.org

Greater Houston Support Group
713-468-4192
Houston@rlsgroups.org

Greater San Antonio RLS Group
210-659-7478
SanAntonio@rlsgroups.org

• Virginia
Central Virginia Support Group
804-273-9900
CentralVirginia@rlsgroups.org

**Fauquier County RLS Support
  Group**
540-364-6138
Fauquier@rlsgroups.org

Lynchburg Area Support Group
434-384-9013
Lynchburg@rslgroups.org

**Northern Virginia RLS Support
  Group**
540-822-4143
NorthernVirginia@rlsgroups.org

Southwest Virginia Support Group
540-544-7454
SWVirginia@rlsgroups.org

**• Washington
Seattle & Vicinity Support Group**
425-881-0163
Seattle@rlsgroups.org

**• West Virginia
Wetzel County WV Support Group**
304-455-2073
WestVirginia@rlsgroups.org

**• Wisconsin
Greater Milwaukee Support Group**
414-964-8185
Milwaukee@rlsgroups.org

Sheybogan RLS Support Group
920-892-7373
Sheybogan@rlsgroups.org

**South Central Wisconsin RLS
  Support Group**
608-276-4002
Madison@rlsgroups.org

West Bend RLS Support Group
920-892-7373
Westbend@rlsgroups.org

**• Cyberspace
Cyber Support Group**
650-747-9252
RLSPLMDWed@rlsgroups.org

INTERNATIONAL

CANADA
Sleep/Wake Disorders Canada
800-387-9253 (in Canada)
416-483-9654
http://swdca.org

**• British Columbia
Okanagan Valley Support Group**
250-549-2280
OkanaganValley@rlsgroups.org

Vancouver Island
250-743-8015
VancouverIsland@rlsgroups.org

• **Ontario**
Brantford Support Group
519-753-1028
Brantford@rlsgroups.org

Hamilton Support Group
905-387-5392
Hamilton@rlsgroups.org

AUSTRALIA
Restless Legs Syndrome Australia
0282-50-60-77
nicc@mail.com
info@rls.org.au

AUSTRIA
RLS Dachverband Österreich
+43664-26-33-100
w.moldaschl@gmx.at
http://www.restless-legs.at/

DENMARK
Restless Legs—Portalen
restless@legs.dk

ENGLAND
Ekbom Support Group
44-(0)-1702-582-002
gill@ekbom-88.demon.co.uk
www.ekbom.org.uk

FINLAND
Levottomat jalat RLSry
(09)-4369-7440
Markku.partinen@rinnekoti.fi
www.uniliitto.fi

FRANCE
AFSJR
02-38-34-32-80
afsjr@wanadoo.fr
www.afsjr.fr

GERMANY
Deutsche Restless Legs
    Vereinigung
089/17-11-18-30
Eisenhome@yahoo.de
www.restless-legs.org

HOLLAND
Zaanstad Stichting Restless Legs
31-20-679-6234
joke.jaarsma@chello.nl
www.stichting-restless-legs.org

JAPAN
Osaka Sleep Health Network
www.oshnet-jp.org

NEW ZEALAND
Nelson—Convenor of Richmond
RLS Support Group
64-3-544-6312
mcrobinson@xtra.co.nz

SPAIN

**Asociación Española de pacientes
con sindrome de piernas
inquietas**

www.aespi.net

SWEDEN

Restless Legs Forbundet

rls@restlesslegs.nu

www.restlesslegs.nu

SWITZERLAND

Restless Legs Switzerland

056-2825403

mathis@insel.ch

auskunft@restless-legs.ch

www.restless-legs.ch

Revised: February 2006

APPENDIX C

Physicians and Researchers

RLSF Medical Advisory Board Members, Past and Present
* indicates current members

David B. Rye, MD, PhD, Chair*
Emory University School of
   Medicine
Atlanta, GA

Charles Adler, MD, PhD*
Mayo Clinic
Scottsdale, AZ

Richard Allen, PhD*
Johns Hopkins Bayview Medical
   Center
Baltimore, MD

Philip M. Becker, MD
Sleep Medicine Institute
Presbyterian Hospital of Dallas

Mark Buchfuhrer, MD, FRCP(C)*
Gallatin Medical Clinic
Downey, CA

David Buchholz, MD
Johns Hopkins University

Sudhansu Chokroverty, MD*
St. Vincent's Hospital
New York, NY

Leslie C. Dinwiddie, RN, MSN

Christopher J. Earley, MD, PhD*
Johns Hopkins Bayview Medical
   Center
Baltimore, MD

Bruce L. Ehrenberg, MD
Tufts New England Medical Center

June M. Fry, MD, PhD

Diego Garcia-Borreguero, MD*
Fundación Jiménez Díaz
Madrid, Spain

Wayne A. Hening, MD, PhD*
New York, NY

Neil Kavey, MD

Clete Kushida, MD, PhD*
Stanford Center of Excellence for
    Sleep Disorders
Stanford, CA

Joseph F. Lipinski Jr., MD

William Ondo, MD
6550 Fannin, Suite 1801
Houston, TX

Barbara Phillips, MD, MSPH
Division of Pulmonary Medicine
Dept. of Medicine
MN 614 UKMC
Lexington, KY

Daniel L. Picchietti, MD

J. Steven Poceta, MD

Frankie Roman, MD

Lawrence Scrima, PhD, ACP

Michael H. Silber, MB, ChB*
Mayo Medical Center
Rochester, MN

Claudia Trenkwalder, MD
Georg-August-Universität
Göttingen, Germany

Arthur S. Walters, MD*
New Jersey Neuroscience Institute
Edison, NJ

Robert Werra, MD*
Ukiah, CA

John Winkelman, MD, PhD*
Sleep Health Center
Newton Center, MA

Marco Zucconi, MD*
H San Raffaele Scientific Institute
Milan, Italy

RLSF Scientific Advisory Board Members, Past and Present
Present members have asterisk by their name.

Allan I. Basbaum, PhD, Chair*
University of California
San Francisco, CA

Bruce Alberts, PhD*
President, National Academy of
  Sciences
Washington, DC

Michael Brownstein, MD, PhD*
National Institute of Mental
  Health
Bethesda, MD

**Marie-Françoise Chesselet,
  MD, PhD***
UCLA School of Medicine
Los Angeles, CA

James R. Connor, PhD*
Penn State College of Medicine
Hershey, PA

Christopher J. Earley, MD, PhD*
Johns Hopkins Bayview Medical
  Center
Baltimore, MD

Steven E. Hyman, MD
Director, National Institute of
  Mental Health

Emmanuel Mignot, MD, PhD*
Associate Professor of Psychiatry and
  Behavioral Sciences
Stanford University
Stanford, CA

William C. Mobley, MD, PhD*
Stanford University
Stanford, CA

**Jacques Montplaisir, MD, PhD,
  CRCPc***
Hôpital du Sacre-Coeur de Montréal
Montréal, Québec
Canada

Pamela Pierce Palmer, MD, PhD*
University of California
San Francisco, CA

Neil Risch, PhD*
Stanford University School of
  Medicine
Stanford, CA

Serge Rossignol, MD, PhD*
Directeur, Centre de recherche en
  sciences neurologiques
Montréal, Québec
Canada

Joseph S. Takahashi, PhD*
Northwestern University
Evanston, IL

Health Care Providers

The RLS Foundation maintains a directory of health care providers who specialize in the treatment of RLS. The following directory has been reprinted with the foundation's permission. (If your area is not listed below, contact the RLS Foundation at 507-287-6465 or visit their website at www.rls.org for names.)

Any decision to use a health care provider from this directory is the sole responsibility of the reader. The listing of these persons does not constitute or imply a recommendation or endorsement by the RLS Foundation, the author, or publisher. By using this directory, the reader assumes full responsibility for use of the information and understands and agrees that the RLS Foundation, author, and publisher are neither responsible nor liable for any claim, loss, or damage from its use. The foundation, author, and publisher disclaim any representation about the directory's accuracy, completeness, or appropriateness for a particular purpose and make no representations concerning the quality of medical care or level of professional skills of any specific health care provider listed.

NAME	CITY	STATE	ZIP	BUSINESS PHONE
Alabama				
William J. Broughton	Mobile	AL	36693	251-660-5757
Gwendolyn C. Claussen	Birmingham	AL	35294	205-975-8116
William J. Hamilton	Mobile	AL	36693	251-660-5108
Joseph Leuschke	Montgomery	AL	36111	334-281-7280
Ann B. McDowell	Dothan	AL	36305	334-793-9564
Stuart J. Padove	Birmingham	AL	35211	205-780-1963
Syed T. Raza	Mobile	AL	36693	251-660-5757
Randy Stubbs	Alexander City	AL	35010	256-215-5602
G. Scott Warner	Cullman	AL	35058	256-739-7050
Alaska				
Anne H. Morris	Anchorage	AK	99508	907-261-3650
Arizona				
Charles H. Adler	Scottsdale	AZ	85259	480-301-8100
Robert Allen	Mesa	AZ	85206	480-981-3000
Mary L. Andrews	Mesa	AZ	85204	480-464-8560
Colin R. Bamford	Tucson	AZ	85724	520-694-8888
Sudeshna Bose	Tucson	AZ	86711	520-694-8053
John N. Caviness	Scottsdale	AZ	85259	none available
Kenneth E. Field	Scottsdale	AZ	85251	602-949-5569
Richard Gilson	Tempe	AZ	85282	480-820-1133
Mohammad A. Kazmi	Lake Havasu City	AZ	86403	928-855-8979
Anthony D. Mosley	Scottsdale	AZ	85258	480-314-2099
Stuart F. Quan	Tucson	AZ	85724	520-694-8888
Johan E. Samantha	Phoenix	AZ	85004	602-406-6315
Ashvin K. Shah	Yuma	AZ	85364	928-344-1891
Holly Shill	Phoenix	AZ	85013	none available
Janet E. Tatman	Scottsdale	AZ	85258	480-905-8755
Michael G. Wade	Mesa	AZ	85206	480-324-0300
Arkansas				
David L. Brown	Fayetteville	AR	72703	501-442-4070
Peggy J. Brown	Searcy	AR	72143	501-278-5610
Paul E. Wylie	Little Rock	AR	72205	501-661-9191

NAME	CITY	STATE	ZIP	BUSINESS PHONE
California				
Eugene Belogorsky	Santa Rosa	CA	95404	707-525-9616
Allan L. Bernstein	Santa Rosa	CA	95403	707-571-4255
Richard A. Beyer	Woodland	CA	95695	530-668-2695
Andrew S. Binder	Santa Barbara	CA	93105	805-898-8845
Reggie Binns	Laguna Hills	CA	92563	877-231-6634
Jed Black	Palo Alto	CA	94304	650-723-6601
Daniel L. Borgstadt	Clovis	CA	93612	none available
Cindy M. Burrell	Los Angeles	CA	90024	818-789-1791
Russell Carter	Manteca	CA	95336	209-239-4554
Wyman Chang	Palo Alto	CA	94304	650-725-7341
Dino Clarizio	Arcadia	CA	91007	616-445-9605
Eric Collins	Oakland	CA	94609	510-834-5778
Emilio L. Cruz	Burbank	CA	91505	818-842-8177
C. Gregory Culberson	San Jose	CA	95119	408-972-6700
Joseph F. Czvik	Vista	CA	92083	760-471-8400
Madeline Schroeder DeCesare	Fresno	CA	93703	559-226-2535
Rajiv K. Dixit	Concord	CA	94520	925-674-2828
Joel Doughten	Riverside	CA	92506	909-682-1622
Mary Kay Dyes	Long Beach	CA	90806	562-490-3580
Robin D. Fross	Hayward	CA	94545	510-784-4607
Yury Furman	Los Angeles	CA	90048	323-782-0160
Asaad Hakim	Garden Grove	CA	92843	714-537-7800
Leonard Hayflick	The Sea Ranch	CA	95497	none available
Neal Hermanowicz	Irvine	CA	92697	714-456-7239
David S. Italleava	West Hollywood	CA	90048	310-652-0920
Richard J. Kanak	Monterey	CA	93940	408-624-8570
Lorne S. Label	Thousand Oaks	CA	91360	805-497-4500
Yuan Yang Lai	North Hills	CA	91343	818-891-7711
Michael A. Lobatz	Encinitas	CA	92024	760-942-1390
Ronald J. Lowell	Daly City	CA	94015	none available
Michael W. Lynch	Fresno	CA	93720	559-229-2786
Kenneth Martinez	Aliso Viejo	CA	92656	949-305-7122
Rafael Pelayo	Stanford	CA	94305	650-723-6601
Norman W. Pincock	Escondido	CA	92025	760-432-6644
J. Steven Poceta	La Jolla	CA	92037	858-554-8895
Ronald A. Popper	Thousand Oaks	CA	91360	805-557-9930
Cheri Quincy	Santa Rosa	CA	95409	707-539-3511
Donald Rebhun	Mission Hills	CA	91345	818-838-4505

NAME	CITY	STATE	ZIP	BUSINESS PHONE
Robert Reyna	Fontana	CA	92335	909-427-4432
Priscilla Sarinas	Palo Alto	CA	94304	650-493-5000
Jon F. Sassin	Santa Rosa	CA	95404	707-525-7616
Paul A. Selecky	Newport Beach	CA	92658	949-760-2070
Renata Shafor	San Diego	CA	92101	619-235-0248
Mark Shapiro	Escondido	CA	92025	760-745-1551
Harold R. Smith	Irvine	CA	92612	949-509-7726
Cheryl L. Spinweber	San Diego	CA	92103	619-260-7378
Steven Suga	Vacaville	CA	95688	707-454-5968
Robert C. Sutter	Laguna Hills	CA	92653	949-837-1133
James P. Sutton	Oxnard	CA	93030	805-278-4148
David M. Swope	Loma Linda	CA	92354	909-558-2880

Colorado

Pinky Agarwal	Englewood	CO	80113	303-788-4600
Robert D. Ballard	Denver	CO	80206	303-398-1523
Marilyn Foelske	Rocky Ford	CO	81067	719-254-7891
Ronald Kramer	Englewood	CO	80110	303-788-4600
Lenore L. Lawson	Brush	CO	80723	970-842-5500
Maureen A. Leehey	Denver	CO	80262	303-315-6456
Steven R. Mohnssen	Colorado Springs	CO	80909	719-471-1069
Lori Moll	Walsenburg	CO	81089	none available
James F. Pagel	Pueblo	CO	81003	719-584-4297
Lawrence Scrima	Aurora	CO	80012	303-671-0977
David I. Slamowitz	Denver	CO	80224	720-200-4884
E. Robert Smith	Denver	CO	80206	303-398-1523

Connecticut

Robert J. DiGiacco	New London	CT	06320	none available
Mahmood Eisa	New Haven	CT	06510	none available
Michael Gauthier	Ridgefield	CT	06877	203-241-8487
Chris Gottschalk	Middletown	CT	06457	860-347-0088
Mohamed N. Hassan	Hartford	CT	06106	860-524-5644
Hellen Kim	Putnam	CT	06260	860-963-2242
John M. Murphy	Danbury	CT	06810	203-748-2551
Charles A. Polnitsky	Woodbury	CT	06798	203-574-6621
Laurence I. Radin	New London	CT	06320	860-443-1891
Dominic Roca	Stamford	CT	06902	203-353-2300
Alan J. Sholomskas	New Haven	CT	06510	203-776-2077
Richard M. Shoup	Manchester	CT	06040	none available

NAME	CITY	STATE	ZIP	BUSINESS PHONE
District of Columbia				
Marshall S. Balish	Washington	DC	20422	202-745-8535
Gregory Belenky	Washington	DC	20307	301-295-7826
Samuel J. Potolicchio	Washington	DC	20037	202-994-4063
David Pruss	Washington	DC	20037	202-833-3000
Perry Richardson	Washington	DC	20037	202-741-2719
Florida				
Ivan F. Ackerman	Brandon	FL	33511	813-655-9000
Glenn D. Adams	Sarasota	FL	34232	941-917-8772
Daniel B. Bell	Saint Petersburg	FL	33701	727-824-7132
William T. Bird	Orlando	FL	32803	407-303-1558
Alejandro D. Chediak	Miami Beach	FL	33140	305-674-2610
Natalio J. Chediak	Boca Raton	FL	33431	561-750-9881
Steven R. Cohen	Saint Petersburg	FL	33701	727-824-7132
Monica Coronel	Hollywood	FL	33021	954-989-6650
Barry Cutler	Pembroke Pines	FL	33027	954-433-0873
John DeCerce	Jacksonville	FL	32209	904-244-9960
Matthew J. Edlund	Sarasota	FL	34239	941-365-4308
Neil T. Feldman	South Pasadena	FL	33707	727-360-0853
Michael F. Finkel	Naples	FL	34119	941-348-4000
Pamela G. Freeman	Orlando	FL	32806	407-859-4540
Ramon A. Gil	Port Charlotte	FL	33952	none available
Timothy L. Grant	Miami	FL	33176	305-595-4041
M. Hanson	Naples	FL	34119	none available
Robert A. Hauser	Tampa	FL	33606	813-844-4077
Charles Henera	Tamarac	FL	33321	954-720-8036
Stuart H. Isaacson	Boca Raton	FL	33486	561-392-1818
Joseph Kaplan	Jacksonville	FL	32224	904-953-2381
V. Daniel Kassicieh	Sarasota	FL	34239	941-955-5858
Jaswinder S. Khara	Sebring	FL	33870	863-471-6600
Lance Kim	Ocala	FL	34474	352-867-9877
Nelson Kraucak	Lady Lake	FL	32159	352-750-4333
Siong-Chi Lin	Jacksonville	FL	32224	904-953-7287
Carlos E. Maas	Port Charlotte	FL	33952	941-613-1777
Nasirdin Madhany	Orlando	FL	32819	407-352-8188
Gauray Malhotra	Spring Hill	FL	34608	352-684-3300
Peter B. McCullagh	Gainesville	FL	32605	352-333-5235
Manuel J. Mier	Venice	FL	34285	none available

NAME	CITY	STATE	ZIP	BUSINESS PHONE
Harold K. Mines	Lakeland	FL	33803	813-680-7271
R. Edward Montejo	Fort Pierce	FL	34950	561-467-0348
Gayle Norris	Pensacola	FL	32501	850-469-7042
Kevin O'Brien	Sumterville	FL	33585	652-793-5900
Gregory J. Piacente	Fort Walton Beach	FL	32547	850-863-8253
Pam Post	Port St. Lucie	FL	34952	772-398-3695
Rammohan S. Rao	Pensacola	FL	32501	850-435-7448
Mitchell S. Rothstein	Jacksonville	FL	32204	904-366-3738
Daniel J. Schwartz	Tampa	FL	33613	813-615-1544
Gregory C. Scott	Saint Petersburg	FL	33701	727-824-7132
David J. Seiden	Pembroke Pines	FL	33026	954-436-2424
Stephen Sergay	Tampa	FL	33609	813-875-5199
William H. Sessions	Orange Park	FL	32073	904-284-8621
David L. Shaw	Niceville	FL	32578	850-269-3930
Robert T. Shebert	Miami	FL	33136	305-243-6732
Carlos Singer	Miami	FL	33136	305-246-6732
R. S. Thornton	Orlando	FL	32803	407-303-1558
Alberto B. Vasquez	Saint Petersburg	FL	33701	727-824-7132

Georgia

John B. Abell	Peachtree City	GA	30269	none available
Jack Blalock	Columbus	GA	31904	706-327-4317
Scott D. Cooper	Canton	GA	30114	770-479-5535
Anthony M. Costrini	Savannah	GA	31419	912-927-5141
Hoyt Crump	Royston	GA	30662	706-245-6177
Mahlon R. DeLong	Atlanta	GA	30322	404-727-3818
Charles M. Epstein	Atlanta	GA	30322	404-778-3440
William T. Garrett	Savannah	GA	31405	912-355-1010
Thomas R. Graff	Albany	GA	31707	229-312-8800
Todd B. Greer	Lawrenceville	GA	30045	none available
Laena Karnstedt	Gainesville	GA	30501	770-297-5013
Randall C. Lanier	Tifton	GA	31794	912-391-4250
David Lesch	Tucker	GA	30084	770-938-3864
Robert A. Pedersen	Dalton	GA	30722	706-275-6121
Hernan Posas	Valdosta	GA	31602	229-242-1234
Frank Puhalovich	Roswell	GA	30076	770-751-1589
David B. Rye	Atlanta	GA	30322	404-727-9825
Jay A. Schecter	Rome	GA	30161	706-236-6343
Kapil D. Sethi	Augusta	GA	30912	706-721-4581

NAME	CITY	STATE	ZIP	BUSINESS PHONE
James J. Wellman	Atlanta	GA	30342	404-257-0080
David Westerman	Atlanta	GA	30342	404-303-1700

Hawaii

Stuart Pang	Honolulu	HI	96819	808-432-7468
Leah L. Ridge	Aiea	HI	96701	808-486-7199

Idaho

John H. Grauke	Moscow	ID	83843	208-882-7565
Beverly J. Ludders	Boise	ID	83704	208-375-8100
Carolyn Rees	Caldwell	ID	83605	206-459-4667

Illinois

J. Steven Arnold	Decatur	IL	62526	217-876-4200
Kenneth S. Aronson	Urbana	IL	61801	217-383-3440
Steven U. Brint	Chicago	IL	60612	312-996-7361
Richard S. Burns	Springfield	IL	62702	217-545-7209
Cynthia L. Comella	Chicago	IL	60612	312-563-2030
Sheryl Coombs	Chicago	IL	60626	773-508-2720
Arif Dalvi	Chicago	IL	60637	773-702-6800
Rodger J. Elble	Springfield	IL	62794	217-545-7182
Arthur W. Fox	Peoria	IL	61603	309-672-5682
Donald A. Greeley	Urbana	IL	61801	none available
Lori M. Guyton	Herrin	IL	62948	618-993-0444
Don Harden	Joliet	IL	60432	888-740-5700
Cathy M. Helgason	Chicago	IL	60612	773-894-5100
Un Kang	Chicago	IL	60637	773-702-6389
W. Bruce Ketel	Glenview	IL	60025	847-294-5490
Ted King	Oak Brook	IL	60523	630-571-0055
Katie Kompoliti	Chicago	IL	60612	312-563-2900
Donald T. Kuhlman	Hoffman Estates	IL	60195	847-882-6604
Steven Lekah	Geneva	IL	60134	630-208-7735
Barry Levy	Des Plaines	IL	60016	847-297-1800
Benjamin D. Margolis	Oak Park	IL	60302	708-383-7899
Charles Martin	Orland Park	IL	60462	708-873-3450
Clifford Massie	Elk Grove Village	IL	60007	none available
D. McDonagh	Schaumburg	IL	60173	847-619-5500
Desmond McDonagh	Chicago	IL	60611	312-642-8346
Nabeela Nasir	Park Ridge	IL	60068	847-723-7024

NAME	CITY	STATE	ZIP	BUSINESS PHONE
Megan A. Nimmers	Rockford	IL	61104	815-489-4429
Kishor Patel	Galesburg	IL	61401	309-344-1000
Sunil A. Patel	Olympia Fields	IL	60461	none available
Daniel L. Picchietti	Urbana	IL	61801	217-383-3100
Ruzica K. Ristanovic	Evanston	IL	60201	847-570-2568
Wayne Rubinstein	Des Plaines	IL	60016	847-298-4088
Muhammad Y. Siddiq	Joliet	IL	60435	815-744-6460
Hai Solomon	Melrose Park	IL	60160	708-450-5090
Jean-Paul C. Spire	Chicago	IL	60637	773-702-6222
V. P. Spire	Chicago	IL	60637	773-702-1780
Suzanne Stevens	Chicago	IL	60612	312-942-5440
Richard Talbert	Maryville	IL	62062	618-288-5711
Evangeline C. Tan	Decatur	IL	62526	217-876-4200
Fred W. Turek	Evanston	IL	60208	847-491-2865
Beth Vilmont	Sterling	IL	61081	815-625-0400
Michael J. Wasserman	Niles	IL	60714	847-298-4590
Barry H. Weber	Park Ridge	IL	60068	847-723-7024
Daniel R. Wynn	Northbrook	IL	60062	847-509-0270
Samuel M. Young	Champaign	IL	61820	217-366-1266

Indiana

NAME	CITY	STATE	ZIP	BUSINESS PHONE
Bradley K. Bittle	Carmel	IN	46032	317-566-0104
Thomas Cartwright	Carmel	IN	46032	317-566-0104
Virgil A. DiBiase	Valparaiso	IN	46383	219-462-1122
Nancy R. Frappier	Kokomo	IN	46901	765-457-4800
Ajay S. Gupta	Bluffton	IN	46714	219-824-3500
John L. Haste	Argos	IN	46501	219-892-5131
Marlin Schul	Indianapolis	IN	46240	317-844-4210
Alan B. Somers	Bloomington	IN	47401	812-334-1242
Naresh Upadhyay	Hammond	IN	46320	219-852-0197
Rajesh Verma	Bluffton	IN	46714	260-824-3500
Thomas Vidic	Elkhart	IN	46514	219-296-3232
Praveen Vohra	Carmel	IN	46032	317-566-0104
Kenneth N. Wiesert	Beech Grove	IN	46107	none available

Iowa

NAME	CITY	STATE	ZIP	BUSINESS PHONE
Todd Ajax	Ames	IA	50010	515-239-4435
Tibor Fulop	Wapello	IA	52653	315-523-8205
Sant Hayreh	Mason City	IA	50401	641-422-6760

NAME	CITY	STATE	ZIP	BUSINESS PHONE
Andrew C. Peterson	Cedar Rapids	IA	52402	319-398-1721
Michael J. Rosenfeld	Grinnell	IA	50112	319-398-1721
Susan E. Sieh	Mason City	IA	50401	none available
Harbhajan Singh	Waterloo	IA	50702	319-272-2600
Donald L. Skinner	Lake City	IA	51449	712-464-3194
Kenneth S. Wayne	Ottumwa	IA	52501	641-682-4594

Kansas

NAME	CITY	STATE	ZIP	BUSINESS PHONE
James A. Cheray	Overland Park	KS	66215	913-541-3340
Gordon R. Kelley	Shawnee Mission	KS	66204	913-384-4200
Kathleen McBratney	Leavenworth	KS	66048	913-651-3111
Leonard Moss	Topeka	KS	66604	785-228-3814
John B. Nelson	Overland Park	KS	66215	913-599-3800

Kentucky

NAME	CITY	STATE	ZIP	BUSINESS PHONE
Gwynne L. Aidala	Glasgow	KY	42141	270-681-1888
Darlene R. Herps	Louisville	KY	40215	502-361-6555
Ken D. McKenney	Bowling Green	KY	42104	877-700-4070
Syed R. Quadri	Radcliff	KY	40160	270-351-3515
John C. Rodrigues	Somerset	KY	42503	606-677-9793
Andrew D. Ruthberg	Lexington	KY	40504	859-258-4450
Jeremiah Suhl	Lexington	KY	40504	859-313-1855
Walter R. Warren	Bowling Green	KY	42101	800-331-9958

Louisiana

NAME	CITY	STATE	ZIP	BUSINESS PHONE
John E. Barrios	New Orleans	LA	70121	504-842-4910
Joseph Y. Bordelon	Opelousas	LA	70570	337-948-7090
Andrew L. Chesson	Shreveport	LA	71130	318-675-5365
Charisse Comeaux	Opelousas	LA	70570	337-943-7146
Gregory S. Ferriss	New Orleans	LA	70115	504-897-4420
Paul A. Guillory	Alexandria	LA	71301	none available
Kevin R. Hargrave	Opelousas	LA	70570	337-942-4567
Kevin R. Hargrave	Lafayette	LA	70506	337-235-4554
Stephen M. Layne	Metairie	LA	70006	504-454-5213
Bruce Lepler	New Orleans	LA	70121	none available
Mary E. McWilliams	Shreveport	LA	71105	318-742-0750
Dhanpat C. Mohnot	Gretna	LA	70056	504-391-7547
Denise Sharon	Baton Rouge	LA	70808	225-766-5656

NAME	CITY	STATE	ZIP	BUSINESS PHONE
Maine				
Roslinde M. Collins	Bangor	ME	04401	207-262-1155
Richard M. Kahn	Auburn	ME	04210	201-784-5489
Maurice Pare	Rangeley	ME	04970	none available
Carl D. Robinsen	Lewiston	ME	04240	207-777-4458
Maryland				
Richard P. Allen	Baltimore	MD	21224	none available
Constance W. Atwell	Bethesda	MD	20892	301-496-9248
William Bara-Jimenez	Bethesda	MD	20892	301-496-1561
F. J. Brinley	Bethesda	MD	20892	301-496-6541
David W. Buchholz	Lutherville	MD	21093	410-583-2830
Tina Byers	Westminster	MD	21157	410-871-7170
Jacques R. Conaway	Baltimore	MD	21237	443-777-8382
Riad Dakheel	Bowie	MD	20716	301-262-0020
Christopher J. Earley	Baltimore	MD	21224	410-550-1044
Helene A. Emsellem	Chevy Chase	MD	20815	301-654-1575
Paul Fishman	Baltimore	MD	21201	410-328-5858
Mark Hallett	Bethesda	MD	20892	301-496-9526
H. A. Jinnah	Baltimore	MD	21287	410-614-6551
Sheppard Kaplow	Towson	MD	21204	410-825-6945
Harry G. Kerasidis	Prince Frederick	MD	20678	410-535-2500
Suzanne Lesage	Baltimore	MD	21224	410-550-2750
Christine Neto	Salisbury	MD	21801	410-546-1001
Natvarlal Rajpara	Westminster	MD	21157	410-840-8100
Stephen G. Reich	Baltimore	MD	21287	410-955-7357
Lisa M. Shulman	Baltimore	MD	21201	410-328-2858
Gordana Stepcic	Berlin	MD	21811	410-641-2220
Camilo Toro	Frederick	MD	21702	301-631-0444
Peter L. Whitesell	Easton	MD	21601	410-822-8930
Massachusetts				
Sanford H. Auerbach	Boston	MA	02118	617-638-8456
Frank P. Calamita	Salem	MA	01970	617-599-4800
Richard Ferber	Boston	MA	02115	617-355-6663
J. Stephen Fink	Boston	MA	02118	617-638-8456
Matthew D. Gold	Newton Lower Falls	MA	02462	617-928-1500
John J. Mooney	Boston	MA	02215	617-632-8405
Yatish M. Patel	Needham	MA	02492	781-455-8924

NAME	CITY	STATE	ZIP	BUSINESS PHONE
Jayant G. Phadke	Worcester	MA	01608	508-363-7300
Charles S. Randall	Newburyport	MA	01950	978-499-7200
Paula D. Ravin	Worcester	MA	01655	508-856-2527
Stacia Sailer	Worcester	MA	01605	508-792-8191
David P. White	Boston	MA	02115	617-527-2227
John W. Winkelman	Newton Center	MA	02459	617-527-2227
Brian Zinsmeister	Lexington	MA	02420	781-862-3953

Michigan

Amer Abarkasm	Roseville	MI	48066	586-771-7440
Loutfi S. Aboussouan	Detroit	MI	48201	313-745-4525
Glen N. Ackerman	Lansing	MI	48912	517-371-3307
R. Obo Addy	Grand Rapids	MI	49546	616-391-3759
Rosa M. Angulo-Kinzler	Ann Arbor	MI	48109	734-647-9851
Gavin I. Awerbuch	Flint	MI	48503	810-733-8338
Shawn L. Bolton	Bloomfield Hills	MI	48304	248-553-0010
Paul A. Cullis	Roseville	MI	48066	586-771-7440
Christopher L. Drake	Detroit	MI	48202	313-916-4455
Bradley K. Evans	Traverse City	MI	49684	231-935-0340
Lisa Ferley	St. Joseph	MI	49085	616-985-0000
Edwin B. George	Detroit	MI	48201	313-745-4275
Sid Gilman	Ann Arbor	MI	48109	none available
Jay M. Gorell	Detroit	MI	48202	313-916-7323
Phillip M. Green	Kalamazoo	MI	49048	none available
Dwayne Griffin	Petoskey	MI	49770	616-487-2100
Gary Gurden	Muskegon	MI	49442	none available
Cassandra M. Klyman	Bloomfield Hills	MI	48302	248-335-7194
Buris Leheta	Roseville	MI	48066	586-771-7440
Carol K. Lyon	Lansing	MI	48912	517-487-2300
Lawrence L. MacDonald	Detroit	MI	48235	313-966-3075
Lee C. Marmion	Grand Rapids	MI	49546	616-391-3759
Margaret L. Moen	Traverse City	MI	49686	231-935-8889
George Mogill	Bloomfield	MI	48304	none available
John H. Morrison	Garden City	MI	48135	734-458-3330
Thomas J. O'Neil	Warren	MI	48093	586-756-5500
Harvey W. Organek	Southfield	MI	48034	none available
Lisa M. Philpot	Tawas City	MI	48763	989-362-0156
Donald B. Reinders	Fremont	MI	49412	231-924-4200
Wendy M. Robertson	Allen Park	MI	48101	313-928-9926

NAME	CITY	STATE	ZIP	BUSINESS PHONE
Gary E. Ruoff	Kalamazoo	MI	49009	616-375-0400
Matthew C. Salon	Traverse City	MI	49684	231-935-0350
Thomas N. Schriefer	Grand Rapids	MI	49525	616-456-9104
Bharat M. Tolia	Bloomfield Township	MI	48302	248-334-0115
Margaret Townsend	Flint	MI	48532	810-733-8338
Richard M. Trosch	Southfield	MI	48034	none available

Minnesota

Janiece Aldinger	Edina	MN	55435	952-920-7200
Chris Armstrong	Edina	MN	55435	952-920-2761
Dana Battles	Minneapolis	MN	55406	none available
Bradley F. Boeve	Rochester	MN	55905	507-284-2511
Scott R. Bundlie	Minneapolis	MN	55415	none available
Joan M. Fox	Orono	MN	55356	612-863-3750
Francisco J. Gomez	Fridley	MN	55432	612-879-1500
Thomas D. Hurwitz	Minneapolis	MN	55417	612-725-2000
Robert G. Jacoby	Fridley	MN	55432	612-879-1500
Keith A. Josephs	Rochester	MN	55905	none available
Suresh Kotagal	Rochester	MN	55905	507-266-0774
Kristin Kuse-Warren	Fairmont	MN	56031	507-238-5025
Mark W. Mahowald	Minneapolis	MN	55415	612-347-6201
Thomas Mulrooney	Woodbury	MN	55125	612-863-3750
Joann V. Neubauer	Willmar	MN	56201	320-231-5005
Wesley Ofstedal	Fosston	MN	56542	none available
John W. Shepard	Rochester	MN	55905	507-284-2511
Michael H. Silber	Rochester	MN	55905	507-284-4032
Shelly Svoboda	Fridley	MN	55432	612-879-1500
Carol J. Winter	Owatonna	MN	55060	507-444-5055

Mississippi

Howard P. Roffwarg	Jackson	MS	39216	601-984-6920

Missouri

Jeffrey L. Belden	Columbia	MO	65201	573-449-0808
John H. Brabson	Springfield	MO	65804	917-820-6525
Roxane S. Bremen	Independence	MO	64057	816-373-3213
A. Cosmo C. Caruso	Kansas City	MO	64114	816-389-6100
Charles D. Donohoe	Independence	MO	64057	816-373-3213
Stephen Duntley	Saint Louis	MO	63108	314-362-4342

NAME	CITY	STATE	ZIP	BUSINESS PHONE
Howard Goldberg	Wentzville	MO	63385	636-332-8482
Shahzad Khan	Columbia	MO	65212	573-882-3133
Amy L. Meoli	Joplin	MO	64804	417-625-2808
Janet E. Morgan	Independence	MO	64055	816-836-4740
Tara M. Nelson	Independence	MO	64057	816-373-3213
Sheryl S. Ream	Arnold	MO	63010	636-464-2888
Curtis Schreiber	Springfield	MO	65807	none available
Oscar A. Schwartz	Creve Coeur	MO	63141	314-878-4699
Todd Silverman	Saint Louis	MO	63141	314-996-8830

Montana

Stephen Johnson	Missoula	MT	59807	406-327-3379
Virginia H. Pascual	Bozeman	MT	59715	406-587-3322

Nebraska

Loretta L. Baca	North Platte	NE	69101	308-534-6687
Teri J. Barkoukis	Omaha	NE	68198	402-559-4087
John Groves	McCook	NE	69001	308-345-4110
Jane McReynolds	Lincoln	NE	68510	402-219-8742
Gilbert Rude	Kearney	NE	68845	308-865-2767
Arthur L. Weaver	Lincoln	NE	68506	402-489-0333

Nevada

Dean L. Mondell	Las Vegas	NV	89144	702-869-5270

New Hampshire

Michele Gaier Rush	Laconia	NH	03246	603-524-3211
Glen P. Greenough	Lebanon	NH	03756	603-650-7534
Sharon Lockwood	Bedford	NH	03110	603-695-2940
Mark A. Lombardo	Concord	NH	03301	603-224-6691
Robert Munger	Exeter	NH	03833	603-773-5200
Carol Pelletier	Nashua	NH	03060	none available
Michele G. Rush	Laconia	NH	03246	603-524-3211
Leslie Suranyi	Laconia	NH	03247	603-524-5151

New Jersey

Mark J. Atkins	Dover	NJ	07801	973-989-3477
Sudhansu Chokroverty	Edison	NJ	08820	732-321-7338
Alan D. Deutsch	Brick	NJ	08724	none available

NAME	CITY	STATE	ZIP	BUSINESS PHONE
Paul Gennaro	West Long Branch	NJ	07764	732-935-1850
David S. Goldstein	Old Bridge	NJ	08857	732-360-4255
Michael G. Kailas	Teaneck	NJ	07666	201-287-0300
Alan S. Lichtbroun	East Brunswick	NJ	08816	732-613-1900
Mangala Nadkarni	West Orange	NJ	07052	972-322-6600
Marc M. Seelagy	Trenton	NJ	08629	609-599-6206
Arthur S. Walters	Edison	NJ	08820	732-321-7000
William D. Wasserstrom	East Brunswick	NJ	08816	732-238-0804

New Mexico

NAME	CITY	STATE	ZIP	BUSINESS PHONE
Marcia Beatty	Taos	NM	87571	505-758-2224
Lee K. Brown	Albuquerque	NM	87102	505-872-6000
Madeleine M. Grigg-Damberger	Albuquerque	NM	87131	505-272-6110
Peter S. Guido	Albuquerque	NM	87109	505-872-6000
Richard Seligman	Albuquerque	NM	87110	505-291-2402

New York

NAME	CITY	STATE	ZIP	BUSINESS PHONE
Timothy Ainslie	Ithaca	NY	14850	607-257-5009
Barbara A. Allis	Huntington	NY	11743	631-351-3815
Ralph J. Ciccone	Staten Island	NY	10306	718-980-5700
Frank Coletta	Freeport	NY	11520	516-379-3139
Lucien Cote	New York	NY	10032	212-305-9173
Leslie D. DiRisio	Rochester	NY	14618	585-442-4141
Lee C. Edmonds	Cooperstown	NY	13326	607-547-3283
David Eidelberg	Manhasset	NY	11030	516-869-9527
Steven Ender	Bethpage	NY	11714	516-520-3962
Stewart A. Factor	Albany	NY	12205	518-452-0914
Stanley Fahn	New York	NY	10032	212-305-5277
Mark F. Gordon	New Hyde Park	NY	11040	718-470-7366
Harly E. Greenberg	New Hyde Park	NY	11040	718-470-7058
Donald S. Higgins	Albany	NY	12205	518-452-0914
Robert Holloway	Rochester	NY	14642	585-275-1018
Lawrence S. Honig	New York	NY	10032	none available
Suzanna Horvath	Brooklyn	NY	11225	718-604-4880
Robert Israel	Rochester	NY	14618	585-442-4141
Thomas M. Kilkenny	Staten Island	NY	10306	718-980-5700
Kiril Kiprovski	New York	NY	10003	212-598-2375
J. M. Kohan	New Hartford	NY	13413	315-798-1652
Stephen A. Kulick	Staten Island	NY	10304	718-448-3210

NAME	CITY	STATE	ZIP	BUSINESS PHONE
Gerard T. Lombardo	Brooklyn	NY	11215	718-780-3017
Jaget S. Mehta	Rochester	NY	14606	585-429-6550
Joseph Modrak	Rochester	NY	14618	585-341-7575
Vinodrai Parmar	Glens Falls	NY	12801	518-793-9155
Anne H. Remmes	New York	NY	10022	212-326-8456
John D. Rogers	New York	NY	10003	212-870-8759
Damon R. Salzman	White Plains	NY	10605	914-997-5751
Joseph P. Santiamo	Staten Island	NY	10312	718-967-3000
Leonid Shkolnik	Brooklyn	NY	11235	718-332-7411
George Silver	Saratoga Springs	NY	12866	none available
C. Stringer	Manlius	NY	13104	315-682-5710
Dhruva G. Sulibhavi	Hicksville	NY	11801	516-733-8000
Michael Thorpy	Bronx	NY	10467	718-920-4891
Andrew P. Tucker	Brooklyn	NY	11215	718-780-5658
Miodrag Velickovic	Yorktown Heights	NY	10598	914-962-5483
Michael D. Weinstein	Mineola	NY	11501	516-663-3907
Nancy Wilcox	Albany	NY	12206	518-689-0206
Rochelle Zak	New Rochelle	NY	10804	914-997-5751
Margarita Zhavoronkova	Rochester	NY	14618	716-442-4141

North Carolina

NAME	CITY	STATE	ZIP	BUSINESS PHONE
Lateef AbuMoussa	Hendersonville	NC	28739	828-694-7630
Kenneth T. Ashkin	Charlotte	NC	28207	704-334-7311
Christopher S. Connelly	Concord	NC	28025	704-262-1911
David H. Cook	Raleigh	NC	27607	909-782-3456
Yvette R. Cook	Cary	NC	27511	919-859-0014
Lindsey E. deGuehery	Wilson	NC	27893	919-291-5864
Alfred A. Demaria	Wilmington	NC	28401	910-341-3358
Michael DiMeo	Burlington	NC	27215	326-538-1234
Julie Draughn	Asheboro	NC	27203	336-629-3500
Kevin C. Gaffney	Salisbury	NC	28144	704-637-3145
Jeannine L. Gingras	Charlotte	NC	28207	704-377-5337
Priscilla Goodwin	Fayetteville	NC	28304	910-323-5288
Stephen C. Hardy	Charlotte	NC	28209	704-377-5337
Keith Hull	Raleigh	NC	27607	919-782-3456
Aatif M. Husain	Durham	NC	27710	919-684-8485
Crystal L. Keith	Rocky Mount	NC	27804	252-443-8221
Kevin M. Klein	Shelby	NC	28150	704-487-7256
William C. Koller	Chapel Hill	NC	27599	919-843-6564

NAME	CITY	STATE	ZIP	BUSINESS PHONE
James D. Mattox	Winston Salem	NC	27103	336-768-8281
A. Thomas T. Perkins	Raleigh	NC	27607	919-782-3456
Rodney A. Radtke	Durham	NC	27710	919-681-3448
Burton L. Scott	Durham	NC	27705	919-668-2493
John G. Steel	Moorehead City	NC	28557	252-726-1083
James S. Wells	Hillsborough	NC	27278	919-967-6353

North Dakota

Joseph Adducci	Williston	ND	58802	701-572-0316
Marjorie E. Henderson	Wahpeton	ND	58075	701-642-2000

Ohio

Anwar Ahmed	Cleveland	OH	44195	216-445-3862
Muhammad I. Akhtar	Portsmouth	OH	45662	740-353-7881
David V. Berkowitz	Cincinnati	OH	45246	513-671-3101
George G. Burton	Kettering	OH	45429	937-395-8805
Robert W. Clark	Columbus	OH	43207	614-443-7800
Cynthia Gaerke	Saint Marys	OH	45885	419-394-9959
Harvey Hanna	Hudson	OH	44236	330-653-5411
Don Higgins	Columbus	OH	43210	614-688-4048
Shahrokh Javaheri	Mason	OH	45040	800-770-7540
Selwyn-Lloyd E. McPherson	Kent	OH	44240	330-673-9641
George W. Paulson	Columbus	OH	43220	none available
Sirg Ramanius	Cleveland	OH	44135	216-267-5933
Marvin H. Rorick	Cincinnati	OH	45242	513-936-5360
Dariush Saghafi	Salem	OH	44460	330-332-7639
Helmut Schmidt	Dublin	OH	43017	614-766-0773
Markus H. Schmidt	Dublin	OH	43017	614-766-0773
Deborah Stouffer	Alliance	OH	44601	330-829-4121
Kingman P. Strohl	Cleveland	OH	44122	216-844-8180
Chang Y. Tsao	Columbus	OH	43205	614-722-4625
Benjamin L. Walter	Cleveland	OH	44195	none available
William S. Wilke	Cleveland	OH	44195	216-444-5624
Virgil D. Wooten	Cincinnati	OH	45220	513-872-4000

Oklahoma

Kersi J. Bharucha	Oklahoma City	OK	73104	405-271-3635
Richard M. Bregman	Tulsa	OK	74136	918-494-1408
Kari A. Casas	Oklahoma City	OK	73104	405-271-8001

NAME	CITY	STATE	ZIP	BUSINESS PHONE
Michael B. Shaw	Tulsa	OK	74133	918-459-8824
Kent R. Smalley	Stillwater	OK	74074	405-377-6378
Ernest Warner	Edmond	OK	73003	405-945-4285

Oregon

Douglas Bailey	Junction City	OR	97448	none available
Gordon Banks	McMinnville	OR	97128	503-474-2722
Bruce Byram	Philomath	OR	97370	none available
Robert W. Crumpacker	Portland	OR	97216	503-256-3034
John J. Greve	Portland	OR	97227	503-288-5201
Valerie Hervey	Albany	OR	97322	none available
Dainis Irbe	Eugene	OR	97401	541-683-3325
Richard A. LaFrance	Corvallis	OR	97330	541-754-1274
Alexandre Lockfeld	Eugene	OR	97401	541-686-2387
Steven D. Maness	Gresham	OR	97030	503-665-9144
Carlos E. Marchini	Grants Pass	OR	97526	541-471-6026
John G. Nutt	Portland	OR	97239	503-494-9054
Noel S. Peterson	Lake Oswego	OR	97034	503-636-2734
Evelyn L. Phillips	Shady Cove	OR	97539	541-878-3730
Gerald B. Rich	Portland	OR	97209	503-228-4414
Norman K. So	Portland	OR	97210	503-229-7246
Deborah R. Syna	Portland	OR	97225	503-291-1422
Robert G. Tearse	Eugene	OR	97041	541-683-3325

Pennsylvania

Sharon Altman	Sharon	PA	15003	724-983-1131
Allison A. Angott	Hermitage	PA	16148	724-981-0825
Mohammad Aslam	Pottsville	PA	17901	570-622-6732
Reena Banka	Philadelphia	PA	19149	215-333-6611
Kevin Booth	Willow Grove	PA	19090	215-957-9250
John F. Brabazon	Ephrata	PA	17522	717-733-2324
David G. Brooks	Philadelphia	PA	19104	215-662-4740
Thomas V. Burke	Williamsport	PA	17701	570-601-1540
Neil A. Busis	Pittsburgh	PA	15232	412-681-2000
Charles R. Cantor	Swarthmore	PA	19081	215-829-6500
John P. Carlson	Danville	PA	17822	570-271-6472
Wissam Chatila	Philadelphia	PA	19140	215-707-5900
Francis Cordova	Philadelphia	PA	19140	215-707-5900
B. Franklin Diamond	Willow Grove	PA	19090	215-957-9250

NAME	CITY	STATE	ZIP	BUSINESS PHONE
John E. Farmer	Waynesboro	PA	17268	717-762-2181
Stanford Feinberg	Wyomissing	PA	19610	610-378-5566
June M. Fry	Lafayette Hill	PA	19444	610-828-4060
Ross N. Futerfas	Allentown	PA	18102	610-821-2826
Irvin M. Gerson	Philadelphia	PA	19137	215-743-4200
Stephen M. Gollomp	Wynnewood	PA	19096	610-642-5371
Constance D. Haber	Monroeville	PA	15146	412-372-7900
Jonathan P. Hosey	Danville	PA	17822	570-271-6590
Thomas C. Hurlbutt	Allentown	PA	18104	610-366-9160
William H. Jeffreys	Danville	PA	17822	570-271-6419
Thomas V. Kantor	Lebanon	PA	17042	717-273-6706
Lawrence A. Kerson	Norristown	PA	19401	610-279-7443
Iqbal Khan	Mountain Top	PA	18707	570-474-6001
Bernadette Krug	Altoona	PA	16602	814-949-4466
George Lapes	York	PA	17403	717-848-3615
Howard J. Lee	Bristol	PA	19007	215-785-9500
Thornton Mason	Philadelphia	PA	19104	215-590-1718
Lydia Murphy-Althouse	Wyomissing	PA	19610	610-378-5566
Clarke U. Piatt	Bryn Mawr	PA	19010	610-672-0104
William R. Pistone	Allentown	PA	18102	610-776-5333
Stacey G. Robert	York	PA	17403	717-851-2521
Anthony Rodriguez	Willow Grove	PA	19090	none available
Denise Rossi	Wyncote	PA	19095	215-886-8452
Michael Shank	Media	PA	19063	610-891-9277
Tanya Simuni	Philadelphia	PA	19107	215-829-7108
Michael J. Soso	Pittsburgh	PA	15213	412-647-9494
Mark M. Stecker	Danville	PA	17822	570-271-6419
Garry Sussman	Perkasie	PA	18944	215-257-0159
John Traveline	Philadelphia	PA	19140	215-707-5900
James Videll	Philadelphia	PA	19152	219-725-7401
Dennis Wayne	Pittsburgh	PA	15224	412-683-7444
Joel B. Younger	Altoona	PA	16602	814-949-3966

Rhode Island

Alice E. Bonitati	Providence	RI	02903	401-444-3567
Carlo Brogna	Westerly	RI	02891	401-596-6207
Joseph H. Friedman	Pawtucket	RI	02860	401-729-2483
Fred F. Griffith	East Providence	RI	02914	401-431-1860
Naomi R. Kramer	Providence	RI	02903	401-831-0611

NAME	CITY	STATE	ZIP	BUSINESS PHONE
Richard P. Millman	Providence	RI	02903	none available
Maria L. Moro-De-Casillas	Pawtucket	RI	02860	401-729-2483
Judith Owens	Providence	RI	02903	401-444-8280

South Carolina

E. M. Alfred	Gaffney	SC	29342	864-489-1446
M. Tariq Ansari	Greenville	SC	29605	864-455-8916
Carol Benoit	Orangeburg	SC	29118	803-536-9818
Richard K. Bogan	Columbia	SC	29201	803-296-5847
Richard G. Leland	Greenville	SC	29615	864-297-6010
Brandon R. Sick	Hartsville	SC	29550	843-383-1624
Wayne B. Sida	Greenwood	SC	29646	864-227-5240
Freddie E. Wilson	Greenville	SC	29607	864-627-5337

Tennessee

Karen Armsey	Knoxville	TN	37917	865-545-7529
Robert L. Cameron	Union City	TN	38261	901-885-5100
Michael L. Eisenstadt	Knoxville	TN	37917	865-545-7529
Michelle Flanagan	Kingsport	TN	37660	423-431-2570
J. Bernard Haynes	Nashville	TN	37205	615-385-1946
William Jurewitz	Fayetteville	TN	37334	931-438-7003
Elizabeth S. Londino	Jackson	TN	38305	731-668-2800
James H. Spruill	Jackson	TN	38301	731-423-1267
John C. Witt	Murfreesboro	TN	37130	615-867-8090

Texas

Philip M. Becker	Dallas	TX	75231	214-750-7776
Kris Bhat	Beaumont	TX	77702	409-835-5382
John R. Burk	Fort Worth	TX	76104	817-336-5864
Ronald D. Cates	Athens	TX	75751	903-675-1717
David R. Duhon	Austin	TX	78746	512-329-9296
Kent T. Ellington	Austin	TX	78731	512-458-6121
Nilgun Giray	Houston	TX	77030	none available
Jamie Grimes	San Antonio	TX	78258	210-916-2203
Kristyna M. Hartse	Dallas	TX	75246	214-820-3200
Joseph Jankovic	Houston	TX	77030	713-798-7438
Sandra L. Knaur	Fort Worth	TX	76104	817-332-7433
Arthur J. Kranz	Dallas	TX	75247	214-638-4801
Cynthia J. Lee	Austin	TX	78758	512-244-1325

NAME	CITY	STATE	ZIP	BUSINESS PHONE
Brian D. Loftus	Houston	TX	77030	713-797-9191
Edgar A. Lucas	Dallas	TX	75246	none available
Prasad Manian	Houston	TX	77030	713-526-5511
Jefy Mathew	The Woodlands	TX	77380	281-296-8788
Claude Mattingly	Jasper	TX	75951	409-384-4621
Adrian Meyer	Richardson	TX	75080	972-231-6341
Greg W. Morgan	Austin	TX	78745	512-558-7770
Byron Myers	Austin	TX	78746	512-329-9296
William G. Ondo	Houston	TX	77030	713-798-7438
David Ostransky	Fort Worth	TX	76107	817-731-0230
Eric J. Pappert	San Antonio	TX	78217	512-558-7770
Raymond Perkins	Tyler	TX	75701	903-592-6907
Kerim F. Razack	Fort Worth	TX	76104	817-332-7433
Rebecca S. Shank	Fort Worth	TX	76132	817-346-5920
Ather Siddiqi	Spring	TX	77380	281-296-8788
Robert R. Springer	Waco	TX	76712	254-741-6767
James M. Stocks	Tyler	TX	75708	903-877-7171
Todd J. Swick	Houston	TX	77024	713-465-9282
Ron Tintner	Houston	TX	77030	713-798-7438
Norma Turk	Houston	TX	77005	713-526-5511
Barbara Weiss	Temple	TX	76508	254-724-5668
Roland Zweighaft	Houston	TX	77024	713-467-8491

Utah

NAME	CITY	STATE	ZIP	BUSINESS PHONE
Evan G. Black	Salt Lake City	UT	84124	801-261-4711
Todd Eberhard	Salt Lake City	UT	84107	801-314-4266
Eric M. Hogenson	Spanish Fork	UT	84660	801-798-7301
Christopher R. Jones	Salt Lake City	UT	84132	801-581-2016
John B. Krugar	Sandy	UT	84094	801-501-2110
David Peterson	Salt Lake City	UT	84106	none available
A. Gordon Smith	Salt Lake City	UT	84132	801-585-6032
Kirk G. Watkins	Saint George	UT	84770	435-634-9630

Vermont

NAME	CITY	STATE	ZIP	BUSINESS PHONE
Christine Connelly	Stowe	VT	05672	802-253-4853
Robert W. Hamill	Burlington	VT	05401	802-847-4589
Keith J. Nagle	Burlington	VT	05401	802-847-2788
Darius Rhodes-Zoroufy	Newport	VT	05855	802-334-4108

NAME	CITY	STATE	ZIP	BUSINESS PHONE
Virginia				
Tom Bond	Williamsburg	VA	23185	757-221-0110
William F. Cale	Harrisonburg	VA	22801	540-434-1721
Debbie Castrinos	Prince George	VA	23875	804-458-5100
John M. Daniel	Richmond	VA	23294	804-346-1515
Simon Fishman	Alexandria	VA	22310	703-313-9111
Seth Greenberg	Virginia Beach	VA	23454	757-481-2515
Rollin James Hawley	Christiansburg	VA	24073	540-731-1627
Antonio S. Jimenez	Fairfax	VA	22031	703-849-8191
Bruce E. Johnson	Virginia Beach	VA	23454	757-481-2515
Vernon H. Kirk	Chesapeake	VA	23320	757-233-2000
Demetrius S. Maoury	Warrenton	VA	20186	none available
Brian J. Mazzei	Abingdon	VA	24210	276-623-0333
Robert W. McMahon	Fishersville	VA	22939	540-332-5878
Julius S. Miller	Chesapeake	VA	23320	757-547-2986
Jacalyn A. Nelson	Danville	VA	24541	434-799-3200
Anthony Quaranta	Virginia Beach	VA	23455	757-363-6850
Baylor Rice	Midlothian	VA	23113	804-897-6447
Hemang Shah	Portsmouth	VA	23703	757-262-0390
Rakesh K. Sood	Richmond	VA	23235	804-323-2255
Joel M. Trugman	Charlottesville	VA	22908	434-243-5931
Kathleen Tylman	Williamsburg	VA	23188	none available
Robert D. Vorona	Norfolk	VA	23507	757-668-3322
G. Frederick Wooten	Charlottesville	VA	22908	434-924-8369
Washington				
Eric M. Ball	Walla Walla	WA	99362	509-525-3720
Berdine S. Bender	Spokane	WA	99204	509-624-0111
Scott T. Bonvallet	Bellevue	WA	98004	425-454-2671
Morris B. Chang	Des Moines	WA	98198	none available
William J. DePaso	Seattle	WA	98101	206-625-7180
Valerie Eckley	Ritzville	WA	99169	509-659-1200
David R. Greeley	Spokane	WA	99204	509-458-7720
Geoffrey M. Greenberg	Yakima	WA	98902	800-657-8805
Patrick J. Hogan	Tacoma	WA	98405	253-383-1066
Noel O. Johnson	Edmonds	WA	98026	425-670-9097
William S. Klipper	Kennewick	WA	99336	509-783-1252
Jon C. Kooiker	Olympia	WA	98506	360-456-1122
Christopher Lawrence	Seattle	WA	98104	206-264-2703

NAME	CITY	STATE	ZIP	BUSINESS PHONE
Daniel Loube	Seattle	WA	98122	206-386-2020
Russell Maier	Yakima	WA	98902	509-452-4520
Jamie Mark	Spokane	WA	99204	509-458-7720
Kimberly A. Mebust	Puyallup	WA	98372	253-848-9656
Philip L. Monroe	Spokane	WA	99216	509-928-6434
John Oakland	Oak Harbor	WA	98277	360-675-8700
Richard Rynes	University Place	WA	98466	253-581-1091
Howard Schaengold	Sammamish	WA	98074	425-868-3338
Sarah E. Stolz	Seattle	WA	98122	206-386-2020

West Virginia

M. Barry Louden	Parkersburg	WV	26104	304-485-5041
Michael A. Morehead	Parkersburg	WV	26104	304-485-5041

Wisconsin

Steven Barczi	Madison	WI	53705	none available
Gerald K. Bayer	Green Bay	WI	54307	920-432-6049
Robert M. Cook	Janesville	WI	53545	608-756-6858
Marco Dotti	Stevens Point	WI	54481	715-346-5050
Jeffrey B. Gorelick	Wauwatosa	WI	53213	414-771-2707
Alfred M. Habel	Kenosha	WI	53143	262-653-5360
Brian M. Hagan	La Crosse	WI	54601	608-782-7300
Kathryn Howells	La Crosse	WI	54601	none available
Sean A. Jochims	Waukesha	WI	53188	262-542-9503
John C. Jones	Madison	WI	53792	608-263-2387
Robert W. Jones	Kenosha	WI	53141	262-656-8888
Michael Katzoff	Milwaukee	WI	53215	414-649-5288
Mary Klink	Madison	WI	53715	608-267-5938
Arne Lagus	Saint Croix Falls	WI	54024	none available
Mark E. Lanser	Janesville	WI	53547	608-755-3522
Lisa Lowndes	Madison	WI	53705	none available
Kathryn L. Middleton	Madison	WI	53715	608-252-8254
Christine Miller	La Crosse	WI	54601	none available
Robert G. Pamenter	Plymouth	WI	53073	920-892-7373
Steven Price	Neenah	WI	54956	none available
Edward P. Vanbeek	Green Bay	WI	54311	920-469-5522

Canada

NAME	CITY	PROVINCE	ZIP	BUSINESS PHONE
Alberta				
Adam Moscovitch	Calgary	AB	T2X 2A8	403-254-6400
British Columbia				
C. Froese	Vancouver	BC	V6T 2B5	604-822-7606
William M. Lemiski	Vernon	BC	V1T 2L5	250-545-1329
Manitoba				
Douglas E. Hobson	Winnipeg	MB	R3C 0N2	204-957-5210
New Brunswick				
Rachel Morehouse	St. John	NB	E2L 4L2	506-648-6174
Nova Scotia				
Malgorzata Rajda	Halifax	NS	B3H 2E2	902-473-4780
Ontario				
John B. Carlile	Kingston	ON	K7L 1S3	613-547-9172
Alan B. Douglass	Ottawa	ON	K12 7K4	613-722-6521
Erwin Feige	North Bay	ON	P1B 7M4	705-472-1967
Raymond Gottschalk	Hamilton	ON	L8P 4M3	905-529-2259
Mark Guttman	Markham	ON	L6B 1C9	905-472-7082
Michael Hawke	Toronto	ON	M4S 1Y2	416-487-1525
Stuart Holtby	Thunder Bay	ON	P7E 6E7	807-622-0333
Lisa Johnston	Toronto	ON	M5T2S8	416-603-5875
Alexander Kunej	Brantford	ON	N3R 2W9	519-752-8100
Anthony E. Lang	Toronto	ON	M5T 2S8	416-603-6422
Clinton Marquardt	Almonte	ON	K0A 1A0	613-255-6906
Lisa Orr	Ottawa	ON	K1Z 7K4	613-722-6521
Colin M. Shapiro	Toronto	ON	M5T 2S8	416-603-5292
Quebec				
Giles Lavigne	Montreal	QC	H3C 3J7	none available
Jacques Montplaisir	Montreal	QC	H4J 1C5	514-338-2693
Eileen Peterson	Montreal	QC	H2X 2K4	514-398-5358

APPENDIX E

Medical Endorsements

Doctors are quoted throughout this book. I have chosen six from different fields and backgrounds to help me introduce Restless Legs Syndrome (RLS), not only to the general public but to doctors and nurses who may never have heard of the affliction.

William C. Dement, MD, PhD, who is sometimes referred to by his peers as "the father of sleep disorders," is author of the often-quoted line "Something has to be done about this terrible disorder. Restless legs syndrome has got to be the biggest completely un-addressed health care priority in America." In the 1950s, Dr. Dement, along with Eugene Aserinsky and Dr. Nathaniel Kleitman, discovered rapid eye movements, or REMs. He is founder and director of the pioneering Sleep Disorders Clinic and Laboratory at Stanford University. He is former chair of the National Commission on Sleep Disorders Research, whose final report led directly to the creation of a new agency within the National Institutes of Health, the National Center on Sleep Disorders Research. He is also former president of the American Sleep Disorders Association, which he helped establish in 1975.

In his book *The Promise of Sleep,* Dr. Dement wrote:

When we founded the world's first sleep disorders clinic at Stanford University in 1970, we tended to see patients whose illness was far advanced. During those early years of clinical activity, I formed the strong opinion that restless legs syndrome was one of the most horrible afflictions I had ever seen. Today, my opinion has not changed, except to accord much more importance to this problem because of its high prevalence. Treatments are available, and with millions of sufferers, there is a great need for a popular book on the subject.

It is disheartening to think of how many people suffer each night from the sometimes tragic consequences of RLS. It is especially disheartening when one realizes that much of this suffering is avoidable. The diagnosis and treatment of sleep disorders like RLS in primary care medicine today is essentially zero.

The lack of awareness is so pervasive that RLS victims don't know what is wrong with them, and doctors don't ask. There is no reason on earth why primary care physicians should not be recognizing the many victims of sleep disorders in their practices.

I urge your readers to help change behaviors or conditions that lead to family dysfunction, workplace accidents, automobile crashes, lost education and income opportunities, disability, and premature death.

Peter Gott, MD, is a general practitioner in Lakeville, Connecticut. He is, in order of importance, our family doctor, a medical columnist syndicated in more than seven hundred newspapers, and author of two books, *No House Calls* and *Getting Off.* His columns on RLS have generated thousands of letters to the RLS Foundation from grateful readers.

To those unfamiliar with the term, "restless legs" sounds like the name of the latest rock group or a TV sitcom. However, to those cursed by the affliction, it's not amusing in any sense of the word. Restless legs syndrome (RLS) is a periodic and predictable descent into Hell. The disorder, of unknown cause, leads to uncontrollable and irresistible leg movements, associated with an unpleasant creeping sensation or unsettled feeling in the lower extremities.

The intensity of restless legs varies from occasional discomfort to nightly crawling sensations that can be relieved only by walking, hence the sobriquet "night-walkers." Although the condition may be associated with a wide range of diseases, such as rheumatoid arthritis and diabetes, most patients are completely healthy. RLS usually worsens with age. It is difficult to describe or treat; consequently, for many sufferers, sleep deprivation and depression are common. Some severely sleep-deprived patients even contemplate suicide.

Most frustrating of all, restless legs syndrome has not been widely recognized by the medical profession. Thus, there are no tests to diagnose it outside of sleep disorder centers, and, for most victims, no consistently effective therapy. Because the syndrome is so underappreciated, patients may be labeled neurotic by their physicians. Also, doctors often confuse restless legs with nocturnal cramps, a different and treatable disorder.

In this valuable book, Robert Yoakum speaks for tormented nightwalkers. As a follow-up to his seminal article in *Modern Maturity* magazine, Yoakum addresses the disorder, validates it, describes the ravages it causes and the research it spawned, and provides the reader with the most current therapy.

Clearly, this is a book that had to be written and is long overdue. It's no surprise that Yoakum, himself a nightwalker, would tackle such a daunting task. A long-standing columnist and observer of the human scene, he brings a welcome freshness to (and detailed analysis of) a puzzling affliction that affects millions. He also brings hope to the sufferers.

Even today, after Yoakum has brought RLS to the attention of the general public via *Modern Maturity*, most doctors and nurses know little or nothing about these disabling disorders.

With at least 10 percent of the population affected, the odds are that every general practitioner has one or more patients with RLS. In most instances the patient will have to live with only a mild case of insomnia, which, even if ignored, will have but little effect on the patient's health and well-being. But for the severely plagued, life may be intolerable. RLS can be as disrupting and debilitating as almost any chronic disease.

An example from my own practice: a woman who, because of her nightly twitches and turmoil, had not slept in the same room with her husband for twenty years read about RLS and asked me about it. I was able to provide a medication that helped—helped enough so that she could again sleep with her partner. It turned out that she had tried, years earlier, to describe the syndrome to me. The difference was that this time around she knew what it was—and so did I.

This book corroborates the reality of a hidden epidemic and affirms the unrecognized anguish caused by restless legs syndrome.

Nightwalkers, you have finally found a voice.

Michael Alderman, MD, is professor in the Department of Epidemiology and Social Medicine at the Albert Einstein College of Medicine and professor of medicine at Cornell University College of Medicine. More than two hundred of Dr. Alderman's articles on health promotion and disease prevention have appeared in the world's leading biomedical journals. He has served as a consultant to the World Health Organization and the U.S. Department of Health and Human Services, as well as New York State and City governments. Past president of the American Society of Hypertension and president of the International Society of Hypertension, he is consultant to the International Rescue Committee and a member of the editorial boards of several medical journals.

In a letter Dr. Alderman wrote,

I was delighted when you decided to write a book on restless legs syndrome. The issue is important. There are millions throughout the world suffering from this fairly intractable and very discomforting condition. As I know, and you have discovered, regrettably few physicians are aware of the problem. Thus, as is usually the case with diseases that haven't yet been fit into neat, well-established categories, most of those who suffer with RLS are unaware that they have an "acceptable" medical problem. The result is unexplained suffering, often in embarrassed and frightening isolation.

Your piece in *Modern Maturity* magazine literally caused an explosion of interest in this heretofore hidden condition and, at the same time, made it possible for patients to describe their problem and seek help. Having an authoritative published piece in hand legitimated their approach to doctors.

I would like to quote Mrs. Pickett Guthrie, founding executive director of the RLS Foundation: "The 'Night Walkers' article was the catalyst that launched our foundation out of obscurity. Without that article, which brought in tens of thousands of letters, we'd still be struggling for recognition in both the medical and lay worlds."

Your book will make a real contribution in two ways. It *will* help millions of people who really suffer. But perhaps of equal importance, it will stimulate the scientific and medical community to explore this common but scientifically challenging ailment.

Victims and the medical community alike should thank you for taking on this very worthwhile task.

Dr. Arthur Walters is founding chair of the Medical Advisory Board of the RLS Foundation, founder of the International RLS Study Group, first recipient of the Ekbom Award, director of the sleep laboratory at New Jersey Neuroscience Institute at JFK Medical Center, and professor in the Department of Neuroscience at Seton Hall University School of Graduate Medical Education.

This book sheds light on restless legs syndrome (RLS), a common but underappreciated disorder characterized by leg discomfort that is worse on lying or sitting and worse at night. Patients complain of strange sensations such as creeping, crawling, tingling, and sometimes pain. Activity provides relief, although in severe cases this is only temporary. Patients devise all sorts of creative strategies to relieve their discomfort, including walking the floor, tossing and turning in bed, leg stretching, leg bending, rubbing their legs, taking hot or cold showers, etc. In most cases patients have difficulty going to sleep and feel the need to walk. In addition, involuntary twitching movements of the legs, called periodic limb movements disorder (PLMD), often disrupt sleep. In severe cases the involuntary leg twitches also occur during wakefulness. Sometimes the arms are involved as well. RLS may develop for unknown reasons; it may run in families or it may develop with nerve damage to the legs from diabetes, kidney failure, or a pinched nerve (sciatica).

RLS was first mentioned in writing three hundred years ago by the great British physician Sir Thomas Willis and only sporadically appears in the literature until the twentieth century. It has been a mere sixty years since the Swede Karl A. Ekbom, MD, more clearly defined the waking symptoms of RLS and a mere forty years since Dr. Elio Lugaresi and colleagues at the University of Bologna, Italy, more clearly characterized the involuntary leg twitches in sleep. Although Ekbom used iron and vasodilators to treat RLS, it is only in recent decades that our modern therapy has evolved to include benzodiazepines, dopamine drugs, anticonvulsants, and opioids.

New frontiers are opening, including the appreciation that RLS occurs more commonly in children than has been heretofore appreciated. Ekbom understood that RLS could be misdiagnosed as growing pains in children, and recent research suggests that RLS can give rise to, or be confounded with, attention-deficit/hyperactivity disorder (ADHD). Jacques Montplaisir, MD, PhD, and his colleagues at the

University of Montreal are using sophisticated electroencephalographic (EEG) techniques to look at the timing of leg sensations, periodic leg movements, and brain waves in order to find the site of nervous system pathology in RLS. Research into the twenty-four-hour variation in symptoms of RLS may lead to biochemical clues as to its cause, and an ongoing multinational search is afoot for the genetic and biochemical basis of hereditary RLS. A U.S.–based nationwide RLS support group network for patients and their families begun in 1992 now claims a database of 65,000 and a regular newsletter. A thirteen-member Medical Advisory Board works closely with the Restless Legs Syndrome Foundation (RLSF) and its support groups. Other distinguished scientists serve on the Scientific Advisory Board. The RLSF has served as a model for similarly based national organizations in other countries. In addition a large International Study Group of prominent physicians and scientists has been formed to work collectively on the RLS problem.

This book details some of this and beyond, but more than anything it gives readers a deeper understanding of the individual and collective suffering, heroism, and sometimes triumph of those whom we serve—our patients.

Wayne Hening, MD, PhD, is a neurologist who has been interested in issues of the motor system and sleep for the past three decades. He began his studies of RLS with Dr. Arthur Walters, a collaboration of the two pioneers that continues to this day. Dr. Hening is now an assistant clinical professor of neurology at UMDNJ–Robert Wood Johnson Medical School. He has been involved in clinical studies and therapeutic trials in RLS as well as epidemiological, circadian, imaging, and genetic studies.

He is currently a coinvestigator in a family study of RLS at Johns Hopkins Bayview Medical Center. Dr. Hening has coauthored over thirty-five original publications in his field of expertise as well as numerous reviews and book chapters. Together with Dr. Walters, he organized the first international symposium on restless legs in 1994. Dr. Hening was one of the earliest members of the Medical Advisory Board of the RLS Foundation and is currently a board member. He serves as secretary of the International RLS Study Group.

June Fry, MD, PhD, former president of the American Sleep Disorders Association, is now director of the Center for Sleep Medicine in Lafayette Hill, Pennsylvania. In an interview, Dr. Fry said:

At the beginning of the last decade it could be said that restless legs syndrome was, as the author's article in *Modern Maturity* magazine described it, "the most common disease you never heard of." But now, finally, RLS is getting the attention its seriousness merits.

RLS victims feel isolated, confused, and misunderstood. That their friends and relatives are now beginning to grasp the gravity of this affliction, and that the medical community is beginning to recognize it as a major sleep disorder, is thanks to the volunteers who launched the RLS Foundation, to the doctors who contributed their skill and time to the cause, to those who funded research, to the journalists who publicized the plight of "nightwalkers," and to the organizers of support groups throughout the nation.

While recent progress in these areas is encouraging, much remains to be done. Certainly the greatest need is for further research into the cause of RLS and into more efficacious methods of treatment. Very little is known, for example, about the genetic factor in RLS. Investigations into its familial nature may shed light on why so many sufferers also experience periodic limb movements disorder (PLMD).

In any event, as is true of the entire field of sleep disorders, scientific knowledge is strength. Obtaining that knowledge will depend on a greater awareness among patients of what they can contribute to their own welfare; on cooperative doctors and nurses; on the willingness of public officials, foundations, and pharmaceutical companies to sponsor research; and on an informed and concerned public. This book will help achieve those urgent goals.

Bruce Alberts, PhD, is president of the National Academy of Sciences and cochair of the RLS Foundation's Scientific Advisory Board.

I have participated in a scientific forum discussing restless legs syndrome and fully support the efforts of the research community to discover the causes of this debilitating disease. This is a serious problem that deserves the attention of some of the nation's best scientists and clinicians, with the goal of developing vastly improved treatments for this puzzling illness.

It is also important to increase awareness of a disease that is too often ignored or misdiagnosed. To that end I encourage your efforts and those of the RLS Foundation.

ACKNOWLEDGMENTS

I am grateful to the editors of *Modern Maturity* magazine, which is now known as *AARP The Magazine*. I might not have written this book had it not been for their willingness to publish my article, "Night Walkers: Do Your Legs Seem to Have a Life of Their Own? Your Torment Has a Name." The editors were surprised and pleased when tens of thousands of readers wrote letters of gratitude and relief at finally seeing their condition described.

I am especially grateful—as any RLS victim should be—to the two hardworking altruists who, in 1992, created the nonprofit RLS Foundation, Pickett Guthrie and Virginia Wilson. Two other pioneers should be mentioned: RLS Foundation president Oron F. Hawley and chair of the board of directors Elmer Hartgerink.

The RLS Foundation was an important source of information. An oasis for RLS victims, the foundation is devoted to "achieving universal awareness, developing effective treatments, and finding a cure." It is the main source of information about RLS for patients and the medical community. It also works with support groups, assists the press, maintains a website (www.rls.org), publishes a quarterly newsletter (*NightWalkers*), answers questions, and provides doctors, nurses, and researchers with a medical bulletin.

Board chairs, who have played key roles in the expanding organization, have been Tim Byrne, 1992–94; Elmer Hartgerink, 1994–96; Sheila Connolly, 1996–99; and Robert Waterman Jr., 2000 to the present. Other dedicated board members, past and present, deserve praise. They include Robert Balkam, Carl G. Belk, Thelma E. Bradt, Martin M. Brinkley, Peter K. Brooks, Marilyn G. Butterfield, Carol Connolly, Willis Daggs, Margarette Fuhr, Mimi Gauthier-LeBien, Pickett M. Guthrie, Frank Gillis, Willard Hayes, Carolyn Hiller, G. Patrick Hunter Jr., Leon Krain, Karen Lazarus, Richard L. Levin, James J. McNichol, Anita Raj, Lester C. Sartorius, Jeanne M. Schell, Gene G. Sivertson, Juanita M. Therrell, Elizabeth L. Tunison, Carol U. Walker, John B. Williams, Virginia N. Wilson, and Diane Wood.

That's a lot of names, but every one of them identifies a person who, early in the search for a cure, contributed to awareness, treatment, and research.

The devotion of board members has been remarkable. They have helped me, each other, and countless RLS victims and their caregivers.

I was especially encouraged and aided by Robert Balkam, past editor of *NightWalkers* and the foundation's able liaison with the federal government.

I also received valuable help from RLS Foundation staff members, particularly Catherine Friederich Murray, former executive director, and Georgianna Bell, present executive director—of all the people I mention, the only ones who are paid. All others work as volunteers, as did founders Guthrie and Wilson. Only a victim can appreciate how much energy these sleep-deprived volunteers needed in order to maintain such an organization. Kathleen and Paul Delage helped me by assisting Virginia Wilson with her book, *Sleep Thief.*

I interviewed dozens of medical professionals in the United States and abroad, each of whom helped expand my understanding of this disease. I attended several conferences where RLS and PLM were on the agenda. I read scores of articles about these diseases in medical journals, not all of which, I admit, I fully understood.

Members of the foundation's Medical Advisory Board were also helpful. The expert on whose crowded schedule I imposed most often was the board's founding chair, Arthur S. Walters, a physician who, along with Richard Allen and Wayne Hening, was a true pioneer, devoting hundreds of hours to research. Joseph Lipinski Jr. was also a source of good advice. Other members (past and present) of that distinguished board, all of whom helped, are Charles Adler, Philip Becker, Mark Buchfuhrer, David Buchholz, Sudhansu Chokroverty,

Lesley C. Dinwiddie, Christopher J. Earley, Bruce Ehrenberg, June Fry, Neil B. Kavey, William Ondo, Ralph Pascualy, Barbara Phillips, Daniel Picchietti, J. Steven Poceta, Frankie Roman, David B. Rye, Lawrence Scrima, Michael Silber, Claudia Trenkwalder, and John Winkelman.

The Scientific Advisory Board also assisted. I am especially indebted to its founding president, Bruce Alberts, and its chair, Allan I. Basbaum. Other members to whom I turned for advice include Michael Brownstein, Marie-Françoise Chesselet, James R. Connor, Steven E. Hyman, Jacques Montplaisir, Pamela Pierce Palmer, Neil Risch, Serge Rossignol, and Joseph S. Takahashi.

Support group organizers and members were an especially welcome source of human-interest stories. I can't list them all here, but I do want to mention Thelma Bradt, the first organizer of the nation's support groups—of which there were very few when I wrote "Night Walkers." There are now nearly a hundred. Elizabeth Tunison, founder of the largest support group, based in Southern California, was a reliable source, as well as her coleader, Barbara Taw. Other helpful sources included Juanita W. Therrell, leader in Bellevue, Washington, and Eileen Gill, who heads the Ekbom Support Group in the United Kingdom.

I am deeply grateful to the busy medical experts who responded to my questionnaires. Virtually every expert in the field, including those in Germany, Italy, Canada, and the United Kingdom—countries in which RLS is now getting the attention it merits—contributed to the book.

No one was more helpful than fellow victims who wrote to share their experiences. I could not, on my testimony alone, have gained the kind of credibility and empathy needed to describe such an enigmatic and devastating affliction. The letters were indispensable in my effort to define the disease for those who haven't had it, and to provide more knowledge and support for those who do. Many letters came from people who responded to that *Modern Maturity* article. Others were sent to the RLS Foundation. I obtained permission to reprint all or part of those letters.

No praise would be adequate for my office associates and first-time editors Kathleen Mahoney, Bonnie Sheldon, and Lisa Brostek, and my wife, Alice, whose patience and concern kept me going at times when, nearly weeping with fatigue and despair, I thought of giving up.

INDEX

ABOUT THE AUTHOR

Robert Yoakum has been a journalist most of his life so it was natural for him, when afflicted with restless legs syndrome, to write about the puzzling disease. His first magazine article on RLS, which carried the subtitle "The most common disease you've never heard of," generated more than 40,000 letters from grateful readers.

Little had been written about RLS, even in medical journals, so the author used his journalistic skills to become an expert. He attended medical conferences, interviewed researchers, and corresponded with other victims.

In his other journalistic life Yoakum wrote a syndicated humor column, worked for Reuters news agency in Paris and for the European edition of the *New York Herald Tribune*, wrote speeches for politicians, one of whom used his phrase, "Eggheads of the world unite, you have nothing to lose but your yolks."